DASH Diet Mediterranean Solution

The Beginner Guide for Weight Loss to Improve Health, includes Meal Prep and Delicious Recipes

By Marla Freeman

Table of Contents

Introduction 1
Chapter 1: The Mediterranean Diet 5
Chapter 2: The DASH Diet 12
Chapter 3: The Mediterranean DASH Diet 17
Chapter 4: Things To Know And Things To Avoid 23
Chapter 5: Food List for the Mediterranean DASH Diet 29
Chapter 6: New Food Terms 32
Chapter 7: Breakfast Recipes 36
   Classic Shakshouka Mediterranean Breakfast 36
   Spinach Mushroom Omelet 38
   Southwest Tofu Scramble 40
   Mediterranean Breakfast Salad 42
   Poached Egg and Salmon on Toast 44
   Mediterranean Eggs 46
   Quinoa and Egg Muffins with Feta 48
   Greek Yogurt Pancakes 50
   Egg White Roasted Tomato Breakfast Sandwich 52
   Baked Eggs with Feta and Avocado 53
   Almond Honey Ricotta with Peaches 54
   Mediterranean Egg Cups 56
   Quinoa Breakfast Bowl 58
   Mediterranean Frittata 60
   Muesli Scones 62

Salmon Cream Cheese Wrap 64

Banana Blueberry Muffins 65

Buckwheat Crepes 67

Blueberry Yogurt Multigrain Pancakes 69

Egg Muffins with Ham 71

Gingerbread Quinoa Bake with Banana 73

Chapter 8: Overnight Oats Recipes 75

Classic oats 75

Chocolate Peanut Butter Oats 76

Carrot Cake 77

Chocolate Coconut 77

Pumpkin Spice 78

Strawberry Cheesecake 79

Tropical fruit 79

Banana Chocolate Chip 80

Apple Cinnamon 81

Berry Oats 81

Chapter 9: Smoothie Recipes 83

Tropical Smoothie 84

Kiwi Smoothie 84

Pineapple Smoothie 85

Melon Smoothie 85

Kale Smoothie 86

Green Smoothie 86

Red Smoothie 86

Avocado Smoothie 87

Beetroot Smoothie 87

Mango Smoothie 88

Chapter 10: Lunch Recipes 89

Halloumi and Herb Tomato Salad 89

Eggplant and Millet Chickpea Stew 91

Chicken and Avocado Salad 93

Cucumber Tomato Toast 95

Greek Chicken and Rice Skillet 96

Mini Chicken Pitas 98

Couscous with Tuna and Pepperoncini 100

Pesto Quinoa Bowls with Roasted Veggies 102

Chicken Salad Stuffed Peppers 104

Stuffed Eggplant 106

Chicken and Farro Salad 108

Pasta with Peppers and Onions 111

Greek Fattoush Salad 112

Tuna and Roasted Pepper Pasta Salad 114

Pomodoro Pasta with White Beans and Olives 116

Pasta alla Erbe 118

Bean Bolognese 120

Florentine Ravioli 122

Macaroni with Sausage and Ricotta 124

Fusilli with Squash and Tomatoes 126

Chapter 11: Soup Recipes 128

Lemon Chicken Soup 128

Greek Spring Soup 130

Moroccan Lentil Soup 132
Roasted Red Pepper and Tomato Soup 134
Mediterranean White Bean Soup 136
Minestrone 138
Dairy-Free Zucchini Soup 140
Tuscan Vegetables Pasta Soup 141
Roasted Cauliflower and Cheddar Soup 143
Meatball Soup 145
White Bean Soup with Sausage and Kale 147
Halibut Chowder 149
Lamb Stew 151
Pasta Faggioli 153
Beef Barley Soup 155
Beef Stew 156
Cabbage and Smoked Sausage Soup 158
Creamy Chicken Tortellini Soup 160
Tuscan Fish Stew 162

Chapter 12: Dinner Recipes 164
Walnut Rosemary Salmon 164
Baked Cod with Maple Mustard 166
Chicken Thighs with Vegetables 168
Almond Artichoke Chicken Breasts 170
Tuna Salad Nicoise 172
Mustard Crusted Salmon Fillets with Roast Cauliflower 174
Roasted Whole Chicken with Lemons and Fennel 176
Caprese Stuffed Portobello Mushrooms 178

Vegetarian Salad Nachos 180
Chicken with Roasted Vegetables and Lemon
    Vinaigrette 182
Chicken with Balsamic Tomato Sauce 185
White Fish with Lemon Orzo 187
Hasselback Caprese Chicken 190
Poached Fish in Basil Tomato Sauce 192
Mediterranean Pasta 194
Chicken Quinoa Bowl 196
Mediterranean Fish en Papillote 198
Feta Chicken Pasta 200
Chicken Parmesan Pasta 202
Tuna Casserole 204
Creamy Tuscan Garlic Spaghetti 206
Zucchini Lasagna Rolls 208
Spicy Salmon with Vegetable Quinoa 210
Shrimp Pasta with Lemon and Garlic 212
Spinach and Feta Macaroni and Cheese 214
Apple Cherry Pork Medallions 216
Black Bean and Sweet Potato Rice Bowl 218
Cod and Asparagus Bake 220
Beef and Blue Cheese Penne with Pesto 221
Pepper Ricotta Primavera 223

Chapter 13: Dessert Recipes 225
Italian Apple Olive Oil Cake 225
Olive Oil Chocolate Chip Cookies 227

Mediterranean Brownies..229

Greek Yogurt Chocolate Mousse 231

Cinnamon Walnut Apple Cake 233

Peanut Butter Banana Greek Yogurt Bowl.................235

Low-Fat Apple Cake 236

Popped Quinoa Crunch Bars 238

Chocolate Olive Oil Cake 240

Maple Vanilla Baked Pears..242

Yogurt with Fresh Strawberries and Honey 243

Tahini and Almond Cookies 244

Pear Cranberry Pie with Oatmeal Streusel 246

Fabulous Fig Bars...248

Strawberry Gelato..250

Chocolate Pistachio Biscotti 251

Almond Cake with Pears 253

Greek Honey Cake 255

Semolina Pudding 257

Chapter 14: Snacks and Appetizers.............................259

Smoked Salmon Feta Cheese Endive Bites................259

Fifteen-Minute Mediterranean Chickpea Salad 260

Loaded Hummus..261

Baked Root Veggies with Parsley Buttermilk Dip.........263

Cucumber Bites with Salmon and Avocado 265

Greek Yogurt Artichoke Spinach Dip 266

Roasted Chickpeas..267

Loaded Eggplant Dip 268

White Bean Artichoke Dip..270
Mediterranean Veggie Fritters...270
Tuna Stuffed Avocados 273
Greek Meatballs..274
Tomato Parmesan Rosemary Palmiers 275
Baby Potatoes with Olive Pesto 276
Herb Cheese Bread 278
Chapter 15: Two Week Meal Plan..279
Chapter 16: The Mediterranean DASH Diet On The Go...284
Conclusion...289

Introduction

In our fast-paced world, it is often very easy to ignore our own health and well-being. We tell ourselves we will worry about it tomorrow. We continuously eat fast food, fat food, and convenience store food in an effort to keep ourselves going. And then one day, we find ourselves overweight, out of shape, and with absolutely no energy to get out of bed in the morning. We want to get healthy, but we don't know where to start. There is more information that we can ever hope to be able to understand.

That is why I created this book *DASH Diet Mediterranean Solution: The Beginner's Guide for Weight Loss to Improve Health, includes Meal Prep and Delicious Recipes* by Marla Freeman. I know it can be confusing in today's busy world to find the right kind of eating plan that will restore us to good health, and we simply don't have time to read every book out there. Well, there is no need to look any further because you've come to the right place.

In this recipe book, you will find everything you need to begin your journey to a healthier lifestyle. Besides having a bit of history to explain where the diet came from, it includes delicious recipes for breakfast, lunch, and dinner. There are also recipes for yummy soups and stews that can actually be served as a complete meal. There are recipes for desserts that won't add inches to your waistline. We will show what food are good foods for the overall diet choices. There is a list of appropriate snack foods.

I've even included a few extras in this book. There is a list of food terms you may not be familiar with and an explanation that tells exactly what they are. One section discusses the mistakes people often make when starting this eating plan. There is a section detailing what foods are consumed on this plan. There is a page that shows pictures of herbs used in cooking these meals. There is also a two-week suggested meal plan created from recipes found in this book.

Overall, this book contains everything you need to get started on a healthier lifestyle with the Mediterranean DASH diet. Read through the book and then give the meal plan a try. Feel free to substitute recipes if you like; the plan is just a suggestion. With all the delicious meal ideas, you will not be disappointed. Happy eating!

Chapter 1: The Mediterranean Diet

It has long been noticed that people who live in those countries that border the Mediterranean Sea tend to live longer and better than most people in America do. They also suffer less from cardiovascular system problems and cancer. This is attributed to living a very active life and enjoying a diet low in saturated fat, sugar, and red meat.

The diet relies heavily on healthy foods such as nuts and produce. The diet may give numerous health benefits such as cancer prevention, brain health, heart health, weight loss, and the prevention and control of diabetes.

There is not one specific 'Mediterranean' diet since there are several countries that have borders on the Mediterranean Ocean. Obvious the Italians, French, Spanish, and Greeks all have very different diets based on food preferences in their own countries. But the basics of their diets are the same.

The basic ideas that make the Mediterranean diet as we know it come from the eating habits of the countries that surround the Mediterranean Sea. In this area olive trees grow abundantly, the mild climate allows fruits and vegetables to be in season year-round, and fish were the gains of the fishermen who could bring home dinner on a daily basis. The many herbs and spices found here were used to flavor food and cure illnesses.

The word "diet" is derived from the Greek word "diaita" which translates to mean "way of life." So, the Mediterranean diet is a way of life and not a diet to be followed for a few months. So by following the Mediterranean diet, we are choosing to follow a healthy eating plan that will give a way of life that will lead to healthy eating and living.

Since the Mediterranean diet has been around for centuries, we can safely say that it may well be the oldest eating plan available in the history of the world. It was recently rediscovered by nutritionists looking for a way to prevent health problems by having people follow a healthy diet plan. It was noted that poor people in small towns in the Mediterranean region were much healthier overall than their wealthier city-dwelling counterparts who had ready access to medical care and a wide variety of food offerings. Further studies verified the researcher's original thoughts that there was a direct link between eating healthy foods and living a healthy lifestyle.

Residents of countries that border the Mediterranean Ocean follow the same basic dietary plan that includes plenty of fruits, vegetables, and fish daily. This diet can reduce the risk of heart disease, high blood pressure, and high cholesterol. Also, people who live in this region have a lower than normal risk of Alzheimer's disease, Parkinson's disease, and cancer.

The Mediterranean Diet is an eating plan and not a specific diet to follow. People using this plan will decide how much weight they want to lose and how many calories they will intake each day. The plan is highly personalized. The pyramid for the Mediterranean diet will help you begin. The items on the pyramid include fish and seafood, legumes, nuts, beans, veggies, and whole grains. The diet puts heavy emphasis on plant-based foods like nuts, legumes, whole grains, vegetables, and fruits. Butter should be used sparingly. Instead, use more canola oil and olive oil. Spices and herbs should be used instead of salt to flavor foods. Fish and poultry should be consumed more often, and red meat limited to a few servings per month. Mealtime should be a time of relaxation and enjoyment and never rushed.

This eating plan also includes one daily glass of red wine. This is not mandatory: we aren't recommending you take up drinking if you don't already! Red wine contains a chemical called resveratrol, an antioxidant chemical that helps protect the body from heart disease and cancer. Resveratrol is also found in grapes, cranberries, and blueberries.

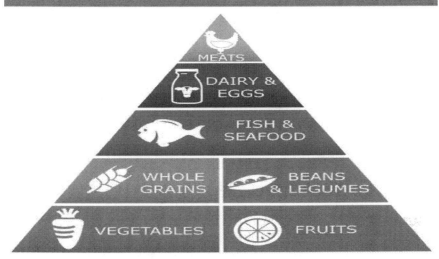

Following the Mediterranean diet does not need to be expensive. Choose fruits and veggies that are on sale. Since less money will be going to buy red meat items that will leave more money for foods that are allowed. The fish, olive oil, and nuts will be more costly, but don't be afraid to check out store brands and other generic brands. They are often the exact same product for half the price. And fish can be bought on sale and frozen. Just make sure it looks fresh when you buy it.

Some people fear that they will gain weight on this diet. It is possible to gain weight on any diet. Weight gain depends on two factors: taking in more calories than are needed and not moving enough to use up those calories as energy. There are plenty of charts on the internet that will give the number of calories needed to lose weight at any current weight.

This is an example of a basic calorie needs chart based on age alone. This chart does not take into account the level of physical activity. Of course, someone who is highly active as an athlete will require more calories daily to be able to perform at their peak. Likewise, someone who sits all day at a desk job will require fewer calories to maintain a healthy weight.

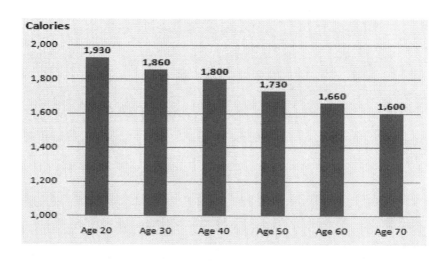

Weight loss is not the primary goal of the Mediterranean diet, but it can easily happen due to the high reliance on plant-based foods. And the foods are high in fiber which will help you feel full for a longer period of time and reduce the possibility of eating too much. Your digestive processes will work better with the introduction of fruits and veggies. The diet can also help people with Type 2 Diabetes control their blood sugar level. All these things are what make the Mediterranean diet a sensible and healthy way to live.

The great success of the Mediterranean diet is found in its great variations of food. It is an eating plan that is known by its dependence on the consumption of eggs, fish, legumes, grains, fruits, and vegetables. It is a traditional diet that will fit well into anyone's lifestyle.

Chapter 2: The DASH Diet

The word DASH, which stands for dietary approaches to stop hypertension, stand for a diet which is purported to lower high blood pressure and help guard against heart disease. The plan is made of the foods we have always been told were good for us to eat, such as grains, veggies, and fruits. These foods contain nutrients that are known to lower blood pressure, such as fiber, calcium, and potassium. DASH also does not encourage foods that are high in salt content or fat content.

After World War II, there has been a steady increase in American in the rates of heart disease and heart-related conditions. The typical American diet is overloaded with saturated fats, too many simple carbohydrates, excessive amounts of Omega Six fatty acids, and too many artificial colors and flavors. In other words, our diets have been processed until they no longer resemble real food. Research into better ways to link diet with overall health resulted in the DASH diet.

The DASH diet leans heavily on vegetables, fruits, and whole grains. Fish and lean poultry are served moderately. Whole wheat flour is used instead of white flour. Using salt is discouraged. Instead, participants are encouraged to season foods with spices and herbs to add flavor without adding salt. DASH as a diet plan promotes the consumption of low-fat dairy, lean meat, fruits, and vegetables. It is literally a mix of old world and new world eating plans. It has been designed to follow old world diet principles to help eliminate new world health problems.

The carbohydrates are mainly made of plant fiber which the body does not easily digest and therefore cannot turn into stored fat. The plan is rich in good fats that make food taste good and help us feel fuller for a longer period of time. Proteins are not forbidden but are geared more toward plant-based protein and not so much meat consumption.

When filling the plate for a meal, it is important that the food be attractive as well as tasty and nutritious. A wide variety of foods will make this plan much more interesting. Try to make choices that will offer a range of colors and textures. And remember that dessert is not off limits but should be based around healthy choices that include fresh fruit.

The DASH eating plans emphasis on vegetables, fruits, whole grains, and low-fat dairy products makes it an ideal plan for anyone looking to gain health through lowered blood pressure and a healthier heart. It is a heart healthy way of eating. The DASH plan has no specialized recipes or food plans. Daily caloric intake depends on a person's activity level and age. People who need to lose weight would naturally eat fewer calories.

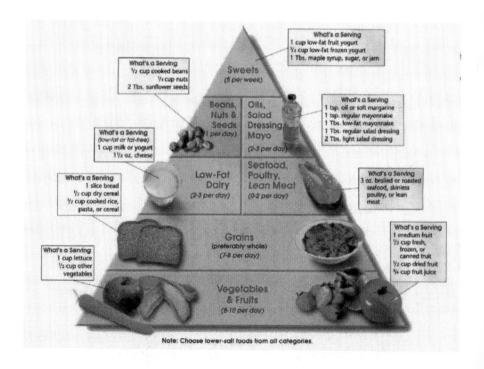

The DASH diet's major focus is on grains, vegetables, and fruits because these foods are higher fiber foods and will make you feel full longer. Whole grains should be consumed six to eight times daily, vegetables four to six servings daily, and fruit four to five servings daily. Low-fat dairy is an important part of the diet and should be eaten two to three times daily. And there should be six or fewer servings daily of fish, poultry, and lean meat. The DASH diet does not limit red meat the way the Mediterranean diet does, but it still keeps it lean.

This is just one of many charts available on the internet that will give a basic caloric count needed to maintain a particular weight or to lose weight. This is just one example.

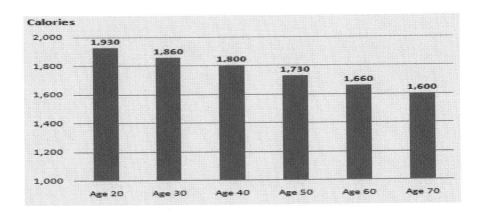

DASH can help control blood pressure that is currently too high and keep it lower in the future. It can also help to avoid heart disease caused by higher than normal blood pressure. The diet can help people lose weight if that is also a goal. And it meets all the daily nutritional needs of the average adult. It is very easy to begin, and it is a diet plan that can transition easily into a lifelong eating plan.

Chapter 3: The Mediterranean DASH Diet

Currently, high blood pressure affects over seventy million people in America. This condition could lead to kidney disease, heart disease, weakening of the arteries, and stroke if it left uncontrolled. Generally, blood pressure readings higher than one forty over ninety are considered high. Besides the people who already have high blood pressure, it is estimated that one American in ever three has prehypertension, which is a condition that can lead to high blood pressure. This is when the blood pressure is higher than 120 over 80. And unfortunately, people can have high blood pressure and not even know it since, in the beginning, it has very few symptoms.

Unfortunately, the average diet is loaded with highly processed food and eating whenever. Research has proven that changes in diet will lead to a healthier lifestyle. These changes include eating a diet that is low in overall sodium and made up of vegetables, fruits, and whole grains. Two of the most popular diets for achieving this new healthy lifestyle are the DASH diet and the Mediterranean diet.

The DASH diet was developed specifically to lower high blood pressure. This plan is proven to cause weight loss and lower blood pressure. It is designed to reduce dependence on sodium in the diet and to promote an increase in the intake of poultry, fish, whole grains, vegetables, and fruits. These foods provide a good source of the nutrients magnesium, calcium, and potassium.

Anyone can follow this diet, so there is no need to make a special diet for one person. The goal of this diet is to promote a healthier lifestyle. There are two plans that have differing levels of sodium intake depending on the recommendations of the doctor. One plan allows for 2300 milligrams per day, and the other plan allows for 1500 milligrams per day.

The Mediterranean diet was originally referred to as the peasant diet because it so closely followed the way people living in the Mediterranean eat. It was developed as a way to fight the growing problem of obesity and the inherent health problems that go with being overweight.

As is the case with the DASH diet, the Mediterranean diet is a complete lifestyle change. The diet encourages consuming more whole foods that are full of nutrients vital to good overall health. It discourages eating foods that are heavily processed or highly refined. Because many different countries have borders on the Mediterranean Ocean, the diet plan includes foods from all of these countries.

There are a few differences between the DASH diet and the Mediterranean diet. They do vary slightly in their recommended intakes of vegetables, fruits, and whole grains each day. The Mediterranean diet is greatly different in the amount of lean meat, fish, and sweets consumed. The DASH diet encourages less dependence on meat and fish than the Mediterranean diet does.

Either diet will provide numerous health benefits for anyone. Both plans, if followed correctly, will lower blood pressure and lead to weight loss. Both plans will reduce the risks associated with cardiovascular disease. Both plans will lower the amount of inflammation in the body. And both plans help to lower the risk of developing diabetes, stroke, heart disease, cancer, and osteoporosis.

So if both of these diets are great by themselves, imagine how they will be when combined in one meal plan. That is the goal of the DASH Diet Mediterranean solution: to combine the two diets together into an awesome diet plan designed to maximize a healthy lifestyle plan. This is a new approach to mix the best of both plans into one delicious diet plan that promotes eating good whole foods and leaving behind the overprocessed fattening foods. Anyone can eat this diet because there are vegetarian meal options along with those featuring meat or fish. It also contains many recipes that are naturally gluten free because they are based on fruits and vegetables.

DASH Diet Mediterranean is a completely safe diet for any member of the family to follow. There is no reason why everyone in the family cannot eat this diet. There is also no reason why anyone would ever need another diet plan because the Mediterranean DASH Solution is really the only diet you will ever need.

These two proven diets come together in an amazing new eating plan that will benefit anyone who tries it. There is a definite link between what kinds of food people eat and how healthy they are. In other words, a healthy diet will lead to a healthy person. And the very foods that the Mediterranean DASH diet is based on are guaranteed to lead to good health. Leafy green vegetables give good amounts of beta carotene and Vitamin K.

Antioxidants come from bright colored veggies. Berries have polyphenols that protect the health of the nerves in the body. Cardiovascular health is supported by whole grains, which also contribute to daily fiber needs. Olive oil is one of the good fats that promote healthy blood flow. Chicken and turkey are more heart-healthy than red meat, although the consumption of red meat is not totally forbidden. Fish is an amazing source of Omega Three fatty acids which promote good brain health and function. Protein is found in beans and lentils, and since they are complex carbohydrates, they keep us feeling fuller longer. And seeds and nuts help reduce the effects of bad cholesterol and high blood pressure.

Following a healthy eating plan consistently is the key to leading a healthier overall lifestyle. And by combining the Mediterranean diet and the DASH diet, you get the best of both worlds. These two diets, when adopted as an overall eating plan, will give the results of a healthy body and a healthy life.

Chapter 4: Things To Know And Things To Avoid

The Mediterranean DASH Diet is a specific eating plan for healthy living, and there are a few things you should know before you begin.

Before going to the grocery store make a list of foods needed for the diet plan. This can be done in two ways. Either make a list based on recipes you want to make or make a generic list of supplies needed and make meals based on the supplies purchased. Whichever method you chose, there are a few important points to keep in mind.

Stay focused on the foods needed to prepare diet-friendly meals. These will be found in the perimeter of the store. A few will be found in the frozen section because frozen vegetables and fish and seafood are acceptable to use. There is nothing in the center of the store needed for these meals.

Buy fresh foods as often as possible. The most daily intake of sodium is found in processed foods, so eliminating these from the diet will help lower the amount of sodium consumed daily. Fresh foods are also lower in fat and sugar. The sugar they do contain is natural food sugar and not the highly processed white sugar that you need to avoid.

Take the time to read food labels. There will be some packaged foods that can be used on this diet, but read the labels and try to avoid excess fats, sugars, and salts.

It is important to fill the kitchen with the staple foods of the Mediterranean DASH diet. Fruits are preferably purchased fresh. Canned fruits should be canned in their own juice, and frozen fruits should be sugar-free. Vegetables can be canned, frozen, or fresh. The canned versions should be without salt added. The frozen ones should not have sauces, butter, or salt added. All dairy products should be low fat. Tortillas, crackers, pasta, rice, cereal, pitas, bagels, and bread should all be the whole grain variety and check the label to buy those that are lower in sodium. Seeds, nuts, and beans should include sunflower seeds, chickpeas (garbanzo beans), lentils, kidney beans, walnuts, and almonds. Always buy the low salt or unsalted variety of the nuts. Look for meats that are lean, and fish and poultry. Chicken and turkey should be skinless. Chose the lean cuts of pork like the tenderloin. Ground beef should be extra lean. Canned meat and fish should be low salt. And try to limit processed or smoked meats.

Olive oil, salsa, flavored vinegar, spices, and herbs can add great flavor to food without the added salt. These may seem to be more costly in the beginning, but they will usually last quite a while since they are used sparingly in recipes.

Cookware that is non-stick is the best because it eliminates the need for added butter or oil for frying and sautéing. This cookware can be found easily without investing a lot of money if you need to purchase a few pieces. A garlic press makes it easier to crush garlic cloves for cooking. Or you can put the clove in a plastic food bag and smash it using a hammer or, if one is available, the flat side of a metal meat tenderizer.

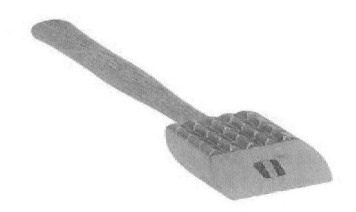

A vegetable steamer is a nice addition to the kitchen since the diet leans heavily on steamed veggies. However, a metal colander set on top of a pot of boiling water and covered with a lid will steam veggies very nicely.

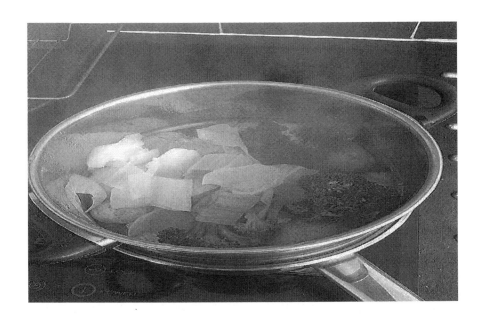

Always rinse canned foods before using. This will help rinse off excess sodium. Don't be afraid to use spices to flavor food. Be careful when using broth because even the low-sodium varieties can have excessive amounts of salt. It is better to make broth from scratch if possible. This is an easy thing to do by boiling chicken for chicken broth or beef for beef broth. A nice veggie broth can be made by boiling the discarded parts of vegetables like the ends and skin of the onion, seeds from bell peppers, carrot tops, celery ends, etc. Put all these items that would usually be thrown away into a large pot and cover them with water. Add some herbs for flavoring. Simmer this mixture two to three hours and strain well. This can be kept in the refrigerator for several days or put in containers and frozen for future use.

Use less meat than you are accustomed to in stews and soups. Use lower fat varieties whenever possible. Mix ground turkey with ground beef to cut most of the fat out of things like hamburgers and meatloaf. And do not feel the need to buy foods you won't eat just because they are in a recipe. Either substitute another item or try a different recipe. There is no sense in making a recipe that is based around avocado if you don't like avocado.

This is a relatively easy and simple diet plan, so there is no need to complicate it with buying special cookware or tools or special foods. Buy simple, fresh foods whenever possible and enjoy!

Chapter 5: Food List for the Mediterranean DASH Diet

While there are no real bad foods, there are foods that are better for good health than others. The foods consumed on the Mediterranean DASH Diet are meant to be fresh, whole, and as healthy as possible to maximize weight loss efforts and allow for healthy eating.

1. Healthy Fats. These are necessary for good health, but they must be of the healthy varieties. Plan on using olive oil, coconut oil, avocados, and avocado oil, and olives, both green and black.

2. Herbs and spices. Get to know and love as many herbs and spices as you can. Bay leaf, cayenne pepper, cinnamon, thyme, turmeric, rosemary, coriander, cloves, garlic, paprika, saffron, ginger, cumin, basil, dill, marjoram, sage, nutmeg, and black pepper.

3. Whole grains. This category includes pasta, oats, buckwheat, couscous, barley, rye, rice, and bread.

4. Legumes. The list of legumes includes lentils, chickpeas, soybeans, peanuts, peas, kidney beans, navy beans, pinto beans, black beans, and butter beans.

5. Seeds and nuts. These help provide healthy fats and proteins to the diet. These include pumpkin seeds, sunflower seeds, cashews, hazelnuts, almonds, and walnuts. If buying them in a jar instead of bulk (like dry roasted) buy the unsalted variety.

6. Fruits and vegetables. Fruits include avocados, melons (all types), berries (passion fruit, kiwi, blueberries, raspberries, blackberries, and strawberries), mangos, bananas, plums, mandarins, nectarines, apricots, grapefruits, oranges, peaches, apples, and pears. Vegetables include tomatoes, onion, shallots, asparagus, celery, yams, and sweet potatoes, red and white potatoes, zucchini, cucumber, squash, pumpkin, broccoli, Brussels sprouts, cabbage, cauliflower, beets, spinach, and lettuce (all varieties).

7. Seafood and fish. Look for all varieties like shrimp, mussels, crab, oysters, salmon, haddock, lobster, tilapia, perch, flounder, and catfish.

These are just suggestions for food items allowed on the Mediterranean DASH diet. The first trip to the grocery store might be rather lengthy while you take the time to learn the items in the perimeter of the store and see what all choices are available.

Chapter 6: New Food Terms

Whenever a new diet plan is started or new recipes are tried, there are always words that make people stop and say "What is that?" So I have included some of the words found in the recipes in this book that may not be familiar to everyone. I just think it helps to know exactly what it is we are eating!

Arborio rice – A short-grained rice that has a higher starch content than most long grain rice.

Balsamic vinegar – A dark vinegar with an intense flavor that originated in Italy. It is made from the whole of the freshly crushed grape—stems, seeds, skin, and juice.

Capers – They are the unopened bud of the flower of the prickly caper plant and are native to the Mediterranean. They have a sharp, salty taste.

Farro – An ancient whole grain similar to quinoa or barley.

Greek yogurt – This yogurt is strained several times until almost all of the liquid has been removed. Its consistency is thicker, its flavor is stronger than regular yogurt, and it has a higher concentration of protein.

Hasselback – This is a technique where a sharp knife is used to cut slits into a food item like meat or a potato to place other foods or herbs into for flavor during cooking. When done correctly the food that has been cut will be fanned out.

Mozzarella pearls – These are bite-sized balls of mozzarella cheese perfect for mixing into sauces or cooking on kebabs.

Orange flower water – This is a natural extract of the orange blossom that infuses the water with the orange flavor and scent.

Peanut butter powder – This powder is made by pressing the oil out of the peanut and then grinding what is left of the nut into a finely ground powder. This resulting powder has the full flavor of peanut butter but eighty-five percent fewer calories from fat than traditional peanut butter.

Pesto – A sauce made with olive oil, Parmesan cheese, garlic, pine nuts, and crushed basil leaves.

Rice vinegar – Also known as rice wine vinegar, it comes from the sugars in rice fermenting into alcohol and then into acid. It is not as acidic as regular white distilled vinegar.

Scallions – A very young green onion.

Shallots – This is a type of onion with a less pungent smell and flavor.

Smoked paprika – The Spanish version of paprika, made from pimiento peppers that are dried, smoked, and ground finely.

Springform pan – This is just a round cake pan with a bottom that is removable. It makes for easier removal of a cake from the pan.

Tahini – A paste made from ground sesame seeds.

Tzatziki – A sauce popular in Greece that is made of cucumbers, garlic, and yogurt.

Whole grain mustard – Prepared mustard with mustard seeds included. Also known as stone ground mustard or coarse ground mustard.

Zest – The rind of a lemon, lime, or orange that is finely grated and used to flavor foods.

Chapter 7: Breakfast Recipes

Classic Shakshouka Mediterranean Breakfast

Prep time ten minutes/cook twenty minutes/serves two to four

Ingredients:

Eggs, four
Chili sauce, one teaspoon
Sugar, one teaspoon
Tomatoes, two cups, chopped
Garlic, two cloves chopped
Red bell peppers, two, shred fine
Onion, one large, shred fine
Salt and pepper, .25 teaspoon each
Olive oil, two tablespoons
Parsley, chopped, one tablespoon

Cook garlic, peppers, and onions five minutes. Mix in sugar, chili sauce, and tomatoes; cook five minutes. Sprinkle with pepper and salt. Make four round spaces and break eggs into spaces. Cook five minutes until eggs set.

Nutrition info: Calories 304, 18.1 grams fat, 623 milligrams sodium, 23.1 grams carbs, 3.8 grams fiber, 1.2 grams sugar, 14.3 grams protein.

Spinach Mushroom Omelet

Prep three minutes/cook fifteen minutes/serves one to two

Ingredients:

Green onion, one, diced
Egg, three
Feta cheese, one ounce
Mushrooms, button, five, sliced
Spinach, fresh, 1.5 cup, chopped
Red onion, .25 cup, diced
Olive oil, one tablespoon

Sauté onions, mushrooms, and spinach for three minutes and set to the side. Beat eggs well and pour into skillet. Let cook three to four minutes until edges begin to brown. Sprinkle all other ingredients onto half the omelet and fold the other half over the ingredients. Cook one minute on each side.

Nutrition info: Calories 337, 25 grams fat, 911 milligrams sodium, 5.4 grams carbs, 1 gram fiber, 1.3 grams sugar, 22 grams protein.

Southwest Tofu Scramble

Prep ten minutes/cook twenty minutes/serves two

Ingredients:

SCRAMBLE

Kale, two cups, chopped
Red pepper, one half, sliced thin
Red onion, one fourth, thin slice
Olive oil, two tablespoons
Eggs, four, beaten

SAUCE

.25 teaspoon turmeric
Chili powder, .25 teaspoon
Cumin powder, .5 teaspoons
Garlic powder, .5 teaspoon
Sea salt, .5 teaspoon
Water, just enough to thin ingredients

Mix spices in a bowl and add just enough water to stir into a sauce consistency. Cook red pepper, onion, and kale for three to four minutes. Pour beaten egg over all and cook until eggs reach desired set.

Nutrition info: Calories 252, 19 grams fat, 516 milligrams sodium, 12.7 grams carbs, 3 grams fiber, 2.5 grams sugar, 12 grams protein.

Mediterranean Breakfast Salad

Prep thirty minutes/serves four

Ingredients:

Lemon, one
Olive oil, two tablespoons
Dill, chopped, .5 cup
Almonds, one cup, chopped
Avocado, one large, sliced
Quinoa, one cup, cooked and cooled
Cucumber, .5, chopped
Tomato, one large in wedges
Arugula, ten cups
Eggs, four, hard-boiled

Mix quinoa, tomatoes, cucumber, and arugula. Add salt, pepper, and olive oil; toss lightly. Place salad on four plates, arrange egg and avocado on top, and then top with almonds and herbs. Drizzle with lemon juice.

Nutrition info: Calories 336, 7.7 grams fat, 946.4 milligrams sodium, 54.6 grams carbs, 5.2 grams fiber, 5.5 grams sugar, 12.3 grams protein.

Poached Egg and Salmon on Toast

Prep ten minutes/cook four minutes/serves two

Ingredients:

Scallions, one tablespoon, thin sliced
Soy sauce, .25 teaspoon
Eggs, two, poached
Salmon, smoked, four ounces
Sea salt and black pepper, .10 teaspoon each
Lemon juice, .25 teaspoon
Avocado, two tablespoons, mashed
Bread, two slices, toasted

Add lemon juice to avocado with salt and pepper. Toast bread and spread avocado mixture over slices. Lay smoked salmon over toast and top with poached egg. Add a splash of soy sauce and top with scallions.

Nutrition info: Calories 389, 17.2 grams fat, 1365 milligrams sodium, 31.5 grams carbs, 9.3 grams fiber, 1.3 grams sugar, 33.5 grams protein.

Mediterranean Eggs

Prep five minutes/cook one hour eighteen minutes/serves six

Ingredients:

Parsley, .25 cup, finely chopped
Sea salt and black pepper
Feta cheese, three ounces
Eggs, eight
Tomatoes, .3 cup, thin slices
Garlic, one clove, chopped
Olive oil, one tablespoon
Butter, one tablespoon
Onion, yellow, one large, thin slices

Cook onions until soft, about ten minutes. Add tomatoes and garlic and cook five minutes. Lower heat and break eggs over the mix, drizzling with pepper, salt, and feta. Cover and cook ten minutes. Sprinkle on parsley and serve.

Nutrition Info: Calories 183, 11 grams carbs, 9 grams protein, 11 grams fat, 255 milligrams sodium, 1 gram fiber, 6 grams sugar.

Quinoa and Egg Muffins with Feta

Prep fifteen minutes/cook thirty minutes/serves six to twelve

Ingredients:

.25 teaspoon salt
Feta cheese, one cup
Quinoa, one cup, cooked
Eggs, eight
Olive oil, two teaspoons
Oregano, fresh chop, one tablespoon
Black olives, .5 cup, chopped
Tomatoes, one cup, chopped
Onion, .5 cup, chopped
Baby spinach, two cups, chopped

Heat oven to 350. Spray oil twelve muffin cup pan. Cook olives, oregano, spinach, tomatoes, and onion five minutes. Beat eggs. Add veggie mix to eggs with cheese and salt. Spoon mix into muffin cups. Bake thirty minutes and keep in the fridge for two days.

Nutrition info one muffin: Calorie 113, 5 grams carbs, 6 grams protein, 7 grams fat, 323 milligrams sodium, 1 gram sugar.

Greek Yogurt Pancakes

Prep fifteen minutes/cook fifteen minutes/serves six

Ingredients:

Blueberries, .5 cup
Milk, .5 cup
Greek yogurt, plain, 1.5 cup
Eggs, three
Butter, three tablespoons
Sugar, .25 cup
Baking soda, one teaspoon
Baking powder, two teaspoons
Salt, .25 teaspoon
Flour, 1.25 cup

Mix dry ingredients and wet ingredients separately, leave blueberries to last. Mix wet and dry ingredients until smooth, then gently fold in blueberries. Top pancakes with more yogurt and blueberries if desired.

Nutrition info six-inch pancake: Calories 73, 1.5 gram fat, 258 milligrams sodium, 8.8 grams carbs, .2 grams fiber, 2.8 grams sugar, 5.6 grams protein.

Egg White Roasted Tomato Breakfast Sandwich

Prep thirty minutes/serves one

Ingredients:

Olive oil, one tablespoon
Grape tomatoes, ten ounces
Provolone cheese, two slices
Ciabatta roll, one
Basil, one teaspoon, chopped
Egg whites, .25 cup
Butter, one teaspoon

Heat oven to 400. Slice tomatoes in half and mix with olive oil. Bake twenty minutes. Cook egg white and place on toasted bread, top with cheese and spice.

Nutrition info: Calories 458, 24 grams fat, 51 grams carbs, 3 grams sugar, 953 milligrams sodium, 2 grams fiber, 21 grams protein.

Baked Eggs with Feta and Avocado

Prep twenty-five minutes/cook fifteen minutes/serves two

Ingredients:

Salt and pepper, .25 teaspoon each
Feta cheese, three tablespoons, crumbled
Olive oil, two tablespoons
Avocado, one large, sliced
Eggs, four

Heat oven to 350. Lay sliced avocado in two oven-safe personal size baking dishes. Crack two eggs in each bowl to not break the yoke. Add cheese crumbles and lightly pepper and salt. Bake fifteen minutes.

Nutrition info: Calories 329, 2.2 grams carbs, 17 grams protein.

Almond Honey Ricotta with Peaches

Prep fifteen minutes/serves four to six

Ingredients:

SPREAD
Honey, one teaspoon
Almond extract, .25 teaspoon
Almonds, .5 cup slice
Ricotta, whole milk, one cup

TO SERVE
Peaches, sliced, one cup
Bread, slice/bagel/English muffin

Mix almond extract, almonds, honey, and ricotta. Spread one tablespoon on toasted bread, cover with peaches.

Nutrition info: Calories 230, 8 grams fat, 90 milligrams sodium, 37 grams carbs, 3 grams fiber, 34 grams sugar, 9 grams protein.

Mediterranean Egg Cups

Prep fifteen minutes/cook twenty-five minutes/serves six

Ingredients:

Bell pepper, 1.5 cups, chopped
Mushrooms, 1.5 cups, chopped
Black pepper, .25 teaspoon
Salt, .10 teaspoon
Garlic powder, .5 teaspoon
Milk, .66 cup
Eggs, ten
Feta cheese, three tablespoons, crumble
Spray oil

Heat oven to 350. Spray oil twelve muffin cup pan. Beat eggs and add pepper, salt, garlic powder, and milk until mixed well. Add in peppers and mushrooms. Fill muffin pan cups with the mix. Bake twenty-five minutes. Cool five minutes then top with cheese and serve.

Nutrition info: Calories 67, 4.7 grams fat, sodium 161.4 milligrams, 1.2 grams carbs, .7 grams sugar, 4.6 grams protein.

Quinoa Breakfast Bowl

Prep thirty minutes/serves six

Ingredients:

Quinoa, two cups, cooked
Feta cheese, one cup
Cherry tomatoes, one pint, cut in halves
Baby spinach, five ounces
Olive oil, one teaspoon
Black pepper, .5 teaspoon
Salt, .5 teaspoon
Garlic, minced, one teaspoon
Greek yogurt, .25 cup, plain
Eggs, twelve

Mix yogurt, salt, pepper, garlic, onion powder, and eggs. Cook tomatoes and spinach five minutes. Add egg mixture and stir until eggs have set to the desired doneness. Mix in quinoa and feta until hot and store in the fridge for two to three days.

Nutrition info: Calories 340, 7.3 grams fat, 30 milligrams sodium, 59.4 grams carbs, 6.2 grams fiber, 21.4 grams sugar, 10.5 grams protein.

Mediterranean Frittata

Prep five minutes/cook twenty minutes/serves six

Ingredients:

Black pepper, .25 teaspoon
Oregano, one teaspoon
Salt, one teaspoon
Feta cheese, .25 cup, crumbled
Black olives, .25 cup, chopped
Green olives, .25 cups
Tomatoes, diced, .25 cup
Milk, .25 cup
Eggs, six

Heat oven to 400. Spray oil an eight in baking dish. Beat milk into eggs and then add other ingredients. Pour into baking dish and bake twenty minutes.

Nutrition info: Calories 107, 7 grams fat, 705 milligrams sodium, 3 grams carbs, 2 grams sugars, 7 grams protein.

Muesli Scones

Prep ten minutes/bake fifteen minutes/serves sixteen

Ingredients:
Honey, two tablespoons
Egg, one
Pistachios, .25 cup, chopped
Sesame seeds, .25 cup
Sunflower seeds, .25 cup
Apricots, dried, chop, .25 cup
Cranberries, dried, .25 cup
Baking soda, .25 teaspoon
Sea salt, .25 teaspoon
Flour, two cups

Heat oven to 350. Mix flour, baking soda, and salt. Add nuts, seeds, and fruits. Whip honey and egg together. Add wet mix to dry, form dough ball. Shape into half-inch thick square shape. Cut in sixteen smaller squares. Bake fifteen minutes.

Nutrition info: Calories 277, 1 gram fat, 58 grams carbs, 8 grams proteins.

Salmon Cream Cheese Wrap

Prep ten minutes/serves two

Ingredients:
Wheat toast, two slices
Basil flakes, .5 teaspoon
Arugula or spinach, .5 cup
Smoked salmon, two ounces
Cream cheese, two tablespoons, low-fat
Red onion, two tablespoons, chopped

Toast wheat bread. Mix basil and cream cheese and spread on toast. Add onion, arugula, and salmon.

Nutrition info: 291 calories, 15.2 grams fat (8.5 saturated), 1101 milligrams sodium, 17.8 grams carbohydrates, 3 grams sugar.

Banana Blueberry Muffins

Prep twenty minutes/cook twenty-five minutes/serves twelve

Ingredients:

Blueberries, fresh or frozen, 1.5 cups
Walnuts, .5 cup, chopped
Baking soda, .5 teaspoon
Sea salt, .5 teaspoon
Cinnamon, 1.5 teaspoon
Baking powder, two teaspoons
Sugar, five tablespoons
Flour, two cups
Canola oil, .25 cup
Vanilla, one teaspoon
Maple syrup, .25 cup
Apple cider vinegar, one teaspoon
Milk, .75 cup + two tablespoons
Mashed ripe banana, .75 cup

Heat oven to 350. Spray oil twelve cup muffin pan. Mix vanilla, maple syrup, vinegar, milk, and bananas. Mix baking soda, salt, cinnamon, baking powder, sugar, and flour in large bowl. Mix wet ingredients into dry. Fold in blueberries and walnuts. Pour batter into muffin cups, bake twenty-five minutes.

Nutrition info one muffin: Calories 180, 5 grams fat, 160 milligrams sodium, 31 grams carbs, 2 grams fiber, 12 grams sugar, 4 grams protein.

Buckwheat Crepes

Prep ten minutes/cook fifteen minutes/serves twelve crepes

Ingredients:

Sugar, one tablespoon
Cinnamon, .25 teaspoon
Canola oil, one tablespoon
Sea salt, pinch
Milk, 1.75 cups,
Flaxseed meal, .75 tablespoon
Flour, one cup

Mix all ingredients until well blended. Pour .25 cup mix into hot skillet while rotating the skillet, so the batter covers all of the bottom thinly. Cook three minutes, flip and cook three more minutes.

Optional fillings include cinnamon apples, warm granola, nut butter, or fruit compote.

Nutrition info without filling: Calories 71, 3 grams fat, 28 milligrams sodium, 8 grams carbs, 1 gram fiber, 1 gram protein.

Blueberry Yogurt Multigrain Pancakes

Prep ten minutes/cook twenty minutes/serves twelve to fourteen pancakes

Ingredients:

Blueberries, fresh, one cup
Salt, .25 teaspoon
Baking powder, one tablespoon + one teaspoon
Sugar, two tablespoons
Barley or rye flour, .25 cup
All-purpose flour, .5 cup
Wheat flour, .5 cup
Vanilla, .5 teaspoons
Lemon zest, .5 teaspoons
Butter, three tablespoons, melted
Milk, four tablespoons
Greek yogurt, plain one cup
Eggs, two

Blend milk, eggs, yogurt, and butter. Mix dry ingredients together. Pour wet into dry and blend. Pour batter into hot skillet .25 cups at a time. Cook three to four minutes each side.

Nutrition info per cake: Calories 98, 3.2 grams fat, 141 milligrams sodium, 15 grams carbs, 1.7 grams fiber, 1.7 grams sugar, 3.1 grams protein.

Egg Muffins with Ham

Prep time ten minutes/cook fifteen minutes/serves six muffins

Ingredients:

Basil, one teaspoon fresh for garnish
Pesto sauce, 1.5 tablespoons
Salt and pepper, .1 teaspoon each
Eggs, six
Feta cheese, .25 cup, crumbled
Spinach, fresh, .3 cup, chopped
Red pepper, roasted, .5 cup
Deli ham, thin slice, nine slices

Heat oven to 400. Spray oil six-cup muffin pan. Place one and one half slice ham in each muffin cup, covering completely. Fill cups with spinach, red pepper, and cheese. Blend salt and pepper with eggs and pour into muffin cups. Bake eighteen to twenty minutes.

Nutrition info one muffin: Calories 109, 6.7 grams fat, 423 milligrams sodium, 1.8 grams carbs, 1.8 grams fiber, 1.2 grams sugar, 9.3 grams protein.

Gingerbread Quinoa Bake with Banana

Prep ten minutes/cook one hour twenty minutes/serves eight

Ingredients:

Almonds, slivered, .25 cup
Milk, 2.5 cups
Quinoa, one cup
Salt, .25 teaspoon
Allspice, ground, .25 teaspoon
Cloves, ground, one teaspoon
Ginger, ground, one teaspoon
Cinnamon, one tablespoon
Maple syrup, .25 cup
Molasses, .25 cup
Bananas, three cups mashed

Heat oven to 350. Spray oil nine by thirteen baking dish. Blend salt, allspice, cloves, ginger, vanilla, cinnamon, maple syrup, molasses, and bananas until smooth. Stir in milk and quinoa. Spoon in the baking dish, bake covered one hour. Uncover, drizzle on sliced almonds, and bake for another twenty minutes.

Nutrition info: Calories 213, 4 grams fat, 41 grams carbs, 18 grams sugar, 211 milligrams sodium, 4 grams fiber, 5 grams protein.

Chapter 8: Overnight Oats Recipes

Sometimes there is just enough time for a quick breakfast and run out the door. These overnight oats recipes are prepared the night before and can be eaten anywhere your busy day takes you. These can be eaten cold or microwaved a few minutes to warm the ingredients. With all recipes, mix all ingredients with oats and spoon into one large container or two smaller containers and refrigerate overnight. Use rolled oats not instant.

Classic oats

Ingredients:

Honey, two tablespoons
Vanilla, .5 teaspoon
Chia seeds, one tablespoon
Milk, .66 cup

Rolled oats, .5 cup

Greek yogurt, .3 cup plain

Chocolate Peanut Butter Oats

Ingredients:

Honey, two tablespoons

Cocoa powder, two tablespoons

Peanut butter, two tablespoons

Vanilla, .5 teaspoon

Chia seeds, one tablespoon

Milk, .66 cup

Rolled oats, .5 cup

Greek yogurt, plain, .3 cup

Carrot Cake

Ingredients:

Cinnamon, ground, .5 teaspoon
Raisins, .25 cup
Cream cheese, two tablespoons room temp
Carrot, one large peel and shred
Honey, two tablespoons
Vanilla, .5 teaspoon
Chia seeds, one tablespoon
Milk, .66 cup
Rolled oats, .5 cup
Greek yogurt, plain, .3 cup

Chocolate Coconut

Ingredients:

Coconut, unsweet flaked, .25 cup
Cocoa powder, two tablespoons

Honey, two tablespoons

Vanilla, .5 teaspoon

Chia seeds, one tablespoon

Milk, .66 cup

Rolled oats, .5 cup

Greek yogurt, .3 cup

Pumpkin Spice

Ingredients:

Nutmeg, ground, .25 teaspoon

Cloves, ground, .25 teaspoon

Cinnamon, .5 teaspoon

Pumpkin puree, plain, .5 cup

Honey, two tablespoons

Vanilla, .5 teaspoon

Chia seeds, one tablespoon

Milk, .66 cup

Rolled oats, .5 cup

Greek yogurt, .3 cup

Strawberry Cheesecake

Ingredients:

Lemon juice, one tablespoon
Cream cheese, three tablespoons, room temp
Strawberries, fresh, .25 cup, chopped
Honey, two tablespoons
Vanilla, .5 teaspoon
Chia seeds, one tablespoon
Milk, .66 cup
Rolled oats, .5 cup
Greek yogurt, plain, .3 cup

Tropical fruit

Ingredients:

Coconut, unsweet flaked
Banana, mashed, one half
Mango, .3 cup, chopped

Pineapple, canned chop .3 cup

Honey, two tablespoons

Vanilla, .5 teaspoon

Chia seeds, one tablespoon

Milk, .66 cup

Rolled oats, .5 cup

Greek yogurt, plain, .3 cup

Banana Chocolate Chip

Ingredients:

Chocolate chips, two tablespoons

Banana, one half, chopped

Honey, two tablespoons

Vanilla, .5 teaspoon

Chia seeds, one tablespoon

Milk, .66 cup

Rolled oats, .5 cup

Greek yogurt, plain, .3 cup

Apple Cinnamon

Ingredients:

Honey, two tablespoons
Cinnamon, ground, one teaspoon
Apples, chopped, .5 cup
Chia seeds, two teaspoons
Milk, .66 cup
Rolled oats, .5 cup

Berry Oats

Ingredients:

Blueberries, .5 cup fresh
Raspberries, .5 cup fresh
Greek yogurt, plain, .5 cup
Milk, .5 cup
Rolled oats, .5 cup

Chapter 9: Smoothie Recipes

Smoothie recipes are a wonderful way to begin any day. Starting the day with a smoothie is a great way to ensure you get enough fruits and veggies in your everyday meal plan. Being rich in vitamins and minerals, they provide much-needed nutrients the body needs for fuel and energy throughout the day.

A delicious smoothie can be made with different fruits and vegetables, and different nuts and spices can easily enhance the taste. A smoothie can be used for a quick breakfast, a replacement meal mid-day, or an afternoon snack to tide you over until dinner.

When using greens, remember to blend them first with a bit of liquid before adding the rest of the ingredients and add any ice last. Fresh fruit is generally preferred, although frozen fruit can help add coldness to the smoothie. Adding drops of lemon juice to the smoothie to preserve freshness allows it to stay fresh in the fridge for two days.

It is best to use whole fruit instead of fruit juice since the same amount of juice usually has about double the calories of the fruit. That, along with the vegetables, the protein, and calcium from milk or yogurt, and the Omega-3 fatty acids from hemp, flax, or chia seeds, makes a smoothie a wonderful way to begin the day.

Tropical Smoothie

Coconut water or milk, .5 cup
Pineapple, fresh, one cup
Mango, one, cubed
Banana, one

Kiwi Smoothie

Basil leaves, one tablespoon
Banana, one

Pineapple, fresh, .5 cup
Kiwi, five

Pineapple Smoothie

Orange juice, .25 cup
Banana, one
Strawberries, .5 cup
Pineapple, fresh, .5 cup

Melon Smoothie

Mint leaves, three
Pear, one
Lemon juice, two tablespoons
Melon, two slices, any type
Cucumber, one half, cubed

Kale Smoothie

Cinnamon, one tablespoon
Apple, one small
Banana, one
Milk, one cup
Kale, leaves, two cups

Green Smoothie

Linseeds, one tablespoon
Banana, one
Cucumber, one small
Lettuce, two leaves
Parsley, one tablespoon
Water, one cup
Spinach, leaves, two cups

Red Smoothie

Linseed oil, one teaspoon
Lemon juice, one tablespoon
Blueberries, .25 cup
Raspberries, .25 cup
Plums, whole chop, three

Avocado Smoothie

Linseeds, one teaspoon
Mint leaves, three fresh
Lime, one
Celery, three stalks
Avocado, one half

Beetroot Smoothie

Pear, one
Carrot, one
Apple, one
Lemon juice, one tablespoon

Ginger, minced, two teaspoons

Beetroot, one, boiled

Mango Smoothie

Mint leaves, fresh, three

Orange, one

Carrot, one

Mango, diced, two cups

Chapter 10: Lunch Recipes

These lunch recipes, besides being delicious, will all travel well, so they are suitable to take to work or school. Or they are great for a brief pause in the middle of any day.

Halloumi and Herb Tomato Salad

Prep ten minutes/serves four

Ingredients:

Basil leaves, five, torn
Olive oil, two tablespoons
Lemon, one half
Parsley, two tablespoons, chopped
Halloumi cheese, .5 pound, sliced
Salt and pepper, .25 teaspoon each
Tomatoes, one pound, sliced

Season tomato slices with salt, pepper, and lemon juice drizzled over. Lay tomatoes on serving plates. Place cheese slices on top of tomatoes and garnish with parsley and basil, then dribble olive oil over all.

Nutrition info: Calories 196, 15 grams fat, 8 grams carbs, 9 grams protein, 6 grams sugar.

Eggplant and Millet Chickpea Stew

Prep thirty minutes/cook ten minutes/serves two

Ingredients:

Hot sauce, two tablespoons
Tomatoes, pureed, one can, fourteen ounces
Onion, one, diced
Eggplant, one, cubed
Salt, .25 teaspoon
Cilantro, two tablespoons garnish
Chickpeas, one can, fourteen ounces, drained
Garlic, three cloves, minced
Black pepper, .25 teaspoon
Olive oil, two tablespoons
Millet, one cup

Bring millet to boil with two cups of water, lower heat and simmer twenty-five minutes; let cool. While millet is simmering, cook onion, garlic, and eggplant with salt and pepper ten minutes. Mix in hot sauce, chickpeas, and tomatoes and cook low for ten minutes. Spoon this mix over millet in bowls.

Nutrition info: Calories 600, 15 grams fat, 100 grams carbs, 20 grams protein, 17 grams sugar.

Chicken and Avocado Salad

Prep thirty-five minutes/cook one hour/serves four

Ingredients:

CHICKEN

Parsley, three tablespoons, freshly chopped

Oregano, one tablespoon, freshly chopped

Olive oil, three tablespoons

Salt and pepper, .25 teaspoon each

Dill, fresh, one tablespoon, chopped

Lemon juice, .25 cup

Lemon zest, one tablespoon

Chicken breast, 1.5 pounds, boneless, skinless

SALAD

Cherry tomatoes, one pint, sliced

Red leaf lettuce, two heads, chopped

Olive oil, .3 cup

Mustard, whole grain, one tablespoon

Broth, chicken, 2.5 cups

Avocados, two, sliced

Onion, red, one, sliced thin

Salt and pepper, .25 teaspoon each

Oregano, dried, one teaspoon

Lemon juice, two tablespoons

Lemon zest, one tablespoon

Barley, one cup

Mix all chicken ingredients except for the chicken into a marinade. Pour over the chicken and refrigerate one hour. Boil broth and barley and lower heat; simmer forty minutes. Fry chicken fifteen minutes each side. Mix tomatoes, onion, and lettuce together and divide into servings. Add barley, avocado slices, and chicken slices to each plate.

Nutrition info: Calories 602, 36 grams fat, 60 grams carbs, 15 grams protein, 8 gram sugar.

Cucumber Tomato Toast

Prep five minutes/serves one

Ingredients:

Balsamic vinegar, one teaspoon
Cream cheese, two teaspoons, whipped
Oregano, dried, .25 teaspoon
Cucumber, one half, diced
Tomato, one half, diced
Whole grain flatbread, two slices
Salt and pepper, .25 teaspoon each
Olive oil, one teaspoon

Mix well the pepper, salt, oregano dill, olive oil, cucumber, and tomato. Spread bread with cream cheese and top with the mix. Drizzle on vinegar to taste.

Nutrition info: Calories 177, 8 grams fat, 24 grams carbs, 3 grams protein, 4 grams sugar.

Greek Chicken and Rice Skillet

Prep fifteen minutes/cook twenty-five minutes/serves four to six

Serve as dinner and take the leftovers to lunch the next day

Ingredients:

Parsley, fresh, .3 cup, chopped
Green olives, one cup
Broth, chicken, 2.5 cups
Garlic, cloves, two, minced
Olive oil, two tablespoons
Garlic powder, one teaspoon
Salt and pepper, .25 teaspoon each
Feta cheese, .25 cup, crumbled
Oregano, fresh, one tablespoon
Rice, long grain, one cup
Red onion, one half, minced
Lemons, three
Oregano, dried, one teaspoon
Chicken thighs, six, boneless, skinless

Heat oven to 375. Salt and pepper chicken thighs. Mix zest from one lemon with garlic powder and dried oregano and cover chicken with this mix. Sear chicken in olive oil five minutes each side. Remove chicken and cook minced garlic and chopped onion five minutes. Then, add rice and cook one more minute. Pour in broth, the juice of the lemon that was zested, and the fresh oregano. Place chicken in ungreased nine by thirteen baking dish and pour rice mixture over the chicken. Bake 25 minutes. Top with lemon slices, fresh parsley, olives, and feta cheese.

Nutrition info: Calories 903, 55 grams fat, 54 grams carbs, 48 grams protein, 5 grams sugar.

Mini Chicken Pitas

Prep one hour ten minutes/cook thirty minutes/serves eight

Ingredients:

CHICKEN
Black pepper, one teaspoon
Coriander, ground, .75 teaspoon
Garlic powder, two teaspoons
Olive oil, .25 cup
Paprika, smoked, .25 teaspoon
Cumin, ground, one teaspoon
Lemon juice, two tablespoons
Lemon zest, one tablespoon
Chicken tenders, one pound

SAUCE
Tomatoes, two, chopped
Romaine lettuce, four leaves, shredded
Salt and pepper, .25 teaspoon each
Parsley, fresh, .25 cup, chopped

Lemon juice, one tablespoon

Cucumber, one half, thin slices

Red onion, one half, thin slices

Dill, fresh, two tablespoons, freshly chopped

Garlic, one clove, grated

Greek yogurt, plain, 1.25 cups

Mini pita bread, sixteen pieces

Mix pepper, paprika, coriander, cumin, garlic powder, lemon juice, lemon zest, and olive oil and pour over chicken in a bowl. Marinate in the refrigerator for one hour. In another bowl mix pepper, salt, dill, parsley, garlic, lemon juice, and yogurt. Refrigerate immediately. Drain marinade and cook chicken five minutes per side. Cut into thin strips. Fill pitas.

Nutrition info per wrap: Chicken: Calories 216, 16 grams fat, 10 grams carbs. 9 grams protein, 0 grams sugar. Sauce: Calories 300, 5 grams fat, 56 grams carbs, 13 grams protein, 4 grams sugar.

Couscous with Tuna and Pepperoncini

Prep three minutes/cook twelve minutes/serves four

Ingredients:

COUSCOUS

Couscous, 1.25 cup

Salt, .75 teaspoon

Broth, chicken, one cup

TUNA MIX

Lemon, one, cut in quarters

Olive oil, to garnish

Parsley, fresh, .3 cup, chopped

Cherry tomatoes, one pint, cut in half

Salt and pepper, .25 teaspoon each

Capers, .25 cup

Pepperoncini, .5 cup slice

Tuna, oil pack, two cans, drained

Boil couscous in broth with salt. Take pot from heat, cover and wait ten minutes. Then loosen grains with a fork. Mix capers, parsley, pepperoncini, tomatoes, and tuna. Serve a scoop of couscous with a scoop of tuna mix, dribble top with olive oil and juice squeezed from a lemon wedge.

Nutrition info: Couscous: Calories 226, 1 gram fat, 44 grams carbs, 8 grams protein, 1 grams sugar. Tuna mix: Calories 193, 9 grams fat, 6 grams carbs, 22 grams protein, 3 grams sugar.

Pesto Quinoa Bowls with Roasted Veggies

Prep ten minutes/cook forty minutes/serves four

Ingredients:

   Parsley, .5 cup, chopped
Garlic, one clove, minced
   Pesto, .5 cup
Salt and black pepper, .25 teaspoon each
Green beans, .5 cup
Zucchini, one medium, cut in cubes
Lemon juice, one tablespoon
Greek yogurt, one cup
Quinoa, one cup
Olive oil
   Cherry tomatoes, one-pint, sliced
Eggplant, one, cut in cubes

Heat oven to 400. Combine beans, cherry tomatoes, zucchini, and eggplant and coat with olive oil. Place on baking pan, bake forty minutes. Boil quinoa with two cups water, lower heat and simmer fifteen minutes.

Loosen grains with a fork. When the quinoa has cooled, add the pesto and mix well. Use a smaller bowl to mix herbs, lemon juice, garlic, and yogurt. Spoon quinoa in four bowls, add veggies around couscous and top with yogurt mix.

Nutrition info: Calories 862, 42 grams fat, 96 grams carbs, 32 grams protein, 23 grams sugar.

Chicken Salad Stuffed Peppers

Prep thirty minutes/cook 0 minutes/serves six

Ingredients:

Cucumber, one half, diced
Scallions, one bunch, sliced
Chicken, cooked, two cups, cubed
Salt and pepper, .25 teaspoon each
Dijon mustard, two tablespoons
Bell peppers, three any color, halved and seeded
Cherry tomatoes, one pint, quartered
Celery, four stalks, sliced
Parsley, .3 cup, chopped
Rice vinegar, two tablespoons
Greek yogurt, .66 cup

Blend parsley, pepper, salt, rice vinegar, mustard, and yogurt. Combine this mix with cucumbers, tomatoes, scallions, celery, and chicken. Spoon chicken mixture into bell pepper halves.

Nutrition info: Calories 116, 3 grams fat, 16 grams carbs, 7 grams protein, 10 grams sugar.

Stuffed Eggplant

Prep ten minutes/cook forty minutes/serves four

Ingredients:

Parsley, fresh chop, three tablespoons to garnish
Salt and pepper, .25 teaspoons each
Thyme, fresh chop, one tablespoon
Kale, two cups, chopped
Garlic, two cloves, minced
Olive oil, three tablespoons, divided
Greek yogurt, plain, .5 cup
Lemon juice, one tablespoon
Lemon zest, one tablespoon
Quinoa, cooked, two cups
Mushrooms, button, one cup, thin slices
Red onion, one, diced
Eggplant, two medium-sized, cut in half

Heat oven to 400. Use a spoon to scoop one-third of eggplant flesh out; save it for another use. Use half of the olive oil to coat eggplant halves and place them on a parchment paper covered baking pan inside facing up. Use the rest of the olive oil to cook garlic, onions, mushrooms, kale, and quinoa for five minutes. Use pepper, salt, lemon juice, lemon zest, and thyme to season this mix. Use the mix to fill eggplant halves and bake for twenty minutes. Sprinkle with parsley and serve sides of yogurt for dipping.

Nutrition info: Calories 339, 15 grams fat, 46 grams carbs, 12 grams protein.

Chicken and Farro Salad

Prep fifteen minutes/cook 40 minutes/serves four

Ingredients:

CHICKEN
Chicken breast, boneless, skinless, one pound, cut into chunks
Olive oil, two tablespoons
Balsamic vinegar, two tablespoons
Dill, fresh, one tablespoon, chopped
Oregano, fresh, one tablespoon, chopped
Paprika, one tablespoon
Garlic, two cloves, minced
   Salt and pepper, .25 teaspoon each
Red potatoes, one pound cut in wedges
Red bell pepper, one, diced
Farro, two cups, cooked
Butter lettuce, one head, torn
Feta, one cup, crumbled
Red onion, cucumber, green and/or black olives, and tzatziki for serving

RED WINE VINAIGRETTE

Olive oil, .25 cup

Red wine vinegar, three tablespoons

Honey, one teaspoon

Lemon juice, two tablespoons

Oregano, fresh, chop, one tablespoon

Garlic, two cloves, minced

Red pepper flakes, crushed, .25 teaspoon

Salt and pepper, .25 teaspoon each

Heat oven to 425. Mix well chicken, salt, pepper, garlic, paprika, oregano, dill, balsamic vinegar, and one tablespoon of the olive oil. Lay chicken in a nine by thirteen baking dish and add bell peppers and potatoes. Bake for forty-five minutes. Blend well all vinaigrette ingredients. Divide lettuce and farro between four bowls and add roasted chicken veggie mix. Drizzle vinaigrette over bowls and serve with tzatziki, olives, and cucumber on the side.

Nutrition info: Calories 782, 3.8 grams fat, 266 milligrams sodium, 19 grams carbs, 4.2 grams fiber, 2 grams sugar.

Pasta with Peppers and Onions

Prep forty minutes/serves four

Ingredients:

Wagon wheel pasta, twelve ounces
Parsley, chop, one tablespoon
Whole peeled tomatoes, one fourteen-ounce can with juice
Red bell pepper, one, chopped
Yellow bell peppers, two, chopped
Crushed red pepper, .25 teaspoon
Salt, .25 teaspoon
Olive oil, three tablespoon
Onion, sweet yellow, 1.5 cups, sliced thin

Cook pasta per package directions. Cook red pepper, onion, and salt in oil in skillet ten minutes. Add in tomatoes and peppers and cook fifteen minutes. Mix in parsley, stirring for one minute, take off heat. Toss with the pasta and serve.

Greek Fattoush Salad

Prep fifteen minutes/cook fifteen minutes/serves four to six

Ingredients:

SALAD
Feta cheese, .75 cup, crumbled
Black olives, .5 cup, sliced
Parsley, fresh, .5 cup, chopped
Red onion, one, small, thin slices
Cherry tomatoes, one cup, sliced
Bell pepper, yellow, chunked
Cucumber, one peeled, quartered and sliced
Romaine lettuce, four cups, chopped
Salt, .25 teaspoon
Olive oil, two tablespoons
Pitas or flatbreads, two whole

DRESSING
Black pepper, .25 teaspoon
Salt, .25 teaspoon

Oregano, .25 teaspoon

Garlic, one clove minced

Red wine vinegar, two tablespoons

Olive oil, .3 cup

Heat oven to 350. Halve the pitas and bake fifteen minutes, turn over once. Break into chunks after cooling. Place chunks in bowl and coat with salt and olive oil. Blend dressing ingredients well in small bowl. Mix olives, parsley, onion, tomatoes, bell pepper, cucumber, and lettuce to large bowl and toss to mix. Add feta cheese, pita bread chunks, and vinaigrette to lettuce mix and toss gently.

Nutrition info: Calories 488, 32.1 grams fat, 1.3 grams sugar.

Tuna and Roasted Pepper Pasta Salad

Prep thirty minutes/serves four

Ingredients:

Whole wheat penne, six ounces
Black pepper, .25 teaspoon
Salt, .25 teaspoon
Garlic, one clove, peeled and minced
Lemon juice, 1.5 teaspoon
Olive oil, one tablespoon
Basil, fresh, two tablespoons
Yogurt, plain nonfat, two tablespoons
Capers, two tablespoons, chopped
Scallions, .5 cup, chopped fine
Roasted red peppers, one jar with seventeen ounces, rinsed and sliced
Tuna, chunk light in water, one six-ounce can

Use package directions to cook pasta, drain and rinse. Mix scallions, capers, half the red peppers, and tuna in a large bowl. Blend well the other half of the red peppers, black pepper, salt, garlic, lemon juice, oil, basil, and yogurt until smooth. Add cooked noodles and sauce mix to tuna mixture and toss well.

Nutrition info: Calories 258, 5 grams fat, 6 grams fiber, 39 grams carbs, 0 grams sugar, 16 grams protein, 476 milligrams sodium.

Pomodoro Pasta with White Beans and Olives

Prep thirty minutes/serves two

Ingredients:

Romano cheese, fresh, grated, two tablespoons
Black pepper, .25 teaspoon
Basil, .fresh, ground, .25 cup
Black olives, two tablespoons chop
Tomatoes, two medium-sized, diced
Garlic, one clove, minced
Cannellini beans, one fifteen-ounce can, drained and rinsed
Olive oil, one tablespoon
Ziti or rigatoni, whole wheat, four ounces

Cook pasta per package instructions. Cook beans and garlic in hot oil five minutes. Take the pan from heat. Add pepper, basil, olives, and tomatoes and mix well.

Place pasta on two plates divided evenly and top with tomato bean mix, sprinkle on cheese and serve.

Nutrition info: Calories 478, 16 grams fat, 14 grams fiber, 74 grams carbs, 21 grams protein, 6 grams sugar, 902 milligrams sodium.

Pasta alla Erbe

Prep forty minutes/serves eight

Ingredients:

Parmesan cheese, fresh, grated, one cup plus one cup for serving
Whole wheat fettuccine, one pound
Tomato paste, two tablespoons
Hot water, one cup
Red pepper, crushed, .25 teaspoon
Salt, 1.25 teaspoon
Garlic, four cloves, peeled and sliced thin
Olive oil, six tablespoons, divided
Leafy greens, beet/chard/spinach, 1.5 pounds, chopped (no stems)

Cook pasta per package instructions. Cook garlic in four tablespoons of oil two minutes. Toss in greens a little at a time, they will begin to wilt and will fit into the pan. Season with crushed pepper and salt and stir well. Cook for about ten minutes. Blend water into tomato paste. Add this to skillet and simmer fifteen minutes. Add cooked pasta to skillet mix and toss well. Pour on one cup of cheese, mix well and serve with another cup for garnish.

Nutrition info: Calories 355, 14 grams fat, 9 grams fiber, 48 grams carbs, 13 grams protein, 3 grams sugar, 566 milligrams sodium.

Bean Bolognese

Prep forty minutes/serves four

Ingredients:

Parmesan cheese, grated, fresh, .5 cup
Fettuccini, whole wheat, eight ounces
Parsley, fresh, chopped, .25 cup, divided
Tomatoes, diced, one fourteen-ounce can
White wine, .5 cup
Bay leaf, one
Garlic, four cloves, peeled and chopped
Salt, .5 salt
Celery, .25 cup, chopped
Carrot, .5 cup, chopped
Onion, one small, chopped
Olive oil, two tablespoons
White beans, one fourteen-ounce can, drained and rinsed

Cook pasta per package directions. Cook celery, carrot, onion, and garlic in oil for ten minutes. Add bay leaf and salt and stir one minute. Remove bay leaf and discard. Pour in wine and boil five minutes. Add beans, tomatoes, and two tablespoons parsley to the skillet and simmer five minutes, stirring often. Spoon pasta into four bowls. Top the pasta with the sauce mix from the skillet. Top with the rest of the parsley and the Parmesan.

Nutrition info: Calories 442, 11 grams fat, 13 grams fiber, 68 grams carbs, 18 grams protein, 9 grams sugar, 766 milligrams sodium.

Florentine Ravioli

Prep twenty minutes/serves four

Ingredients:

Parmesan cheese, fresh grated, .25 cups
Water, .5 cup
Spinach, frozen, sixteen-ounce bag, thawed
Crushed red pepper, .25 teaspoon
Salt, .25 teaspoon
Garlic, four cloves, minced
Olive oil, six teaspoons
Cheese ravioli, frozen, one twenty-ounce package

Cook ravioli per package directions. Cook spinach, red peppers, water, and garlic in hot oil five to eight minutes until spinach thaws and wilts. Divide spinach mix into four bowls and top with the cooked pasta. Garnish with Parmesan cheese.

Nutrition info: Calories 263, 13 grams fat, 5 grams fiber, 29 grams carbs, 12 grams protein, 7 grams sugar, 674 milligrams sodium.

Macaroni with Sausage and Ricotta

Prep thirty five minutes/serves six

Ingredients:

Parmesan cheese, fresh, grated, .25 cup
Basil leaves, fresh, ten, thin slices
Ricotta cheese, part skim, six tablespoons
Elbow macaroni, twelve ounces
Salt, .25 teaspoon and one tablespoon
Black pepper, .25 teaspoon
Whole peeled tomatoes, canned, one fourteen-ounce can with juice
Pork sausage, mild, remove the casing, six ounces
Yellow onion, finely chopped, six tablespoons
Olive oil, two tablespoons

Cook pasta per package directions with one tablespoon salt. Cook sausage and onion in hot oil in skillet five minutes. Add pepper, tomatoes, and .25 teaspoon salt and cook ten minutes. Stir in pasta with basil and ricotta until well mixed. Garnish with Parmesan and serve.

Nutrition info: Calories 361, 12 grams fat, 4 grams fiber, 48 grams carbs, 14 grams protein, 3 grams sugar, 446 milligrams sodium.

Fusilli with Squash and Tomatoes

Prep twenty five minutes/serves six

Ingredients:

Fusilli pasta, twelve ounces
Grape tomatoes, two cups, sliced in half
Black pepper, .25 teaspoon
Salt, .25 teaspoon
Thyme, chop, one tablespoon
Squash, yellow, one pound
Onion, yellow, one, thin slices

Cook pasta per package directions. Cut the neck off the squash. Cut squash into quarters longwise and slice thin. Cook squash, thyme, onion, pepper, and salt in oil ten minutes, stirring often. Pour in tomatoes and cook five more minutes. Add cooked pasta and mix well.

Nutrition info: Calories 311, 9 grams fat, 4 grams fiber, 49 grams carbs, 10 grams proteins, 5 grams sugar, 339 milligrams sodium.

Chapter 11: Soup Recipes

Lemon Chicken Soup

Prep ten minutes/cook twenty minutes/serves six

Ingredients:

Dill, fresh, two tablespoons, chopped
Parsley, two tablespoons, chopped
Lemon juice, two tablespoons
Spinach, baby, four cups
Cannellini beans, two can, 15.5 ounces each, drained and rinsed
Bay leaves, two
Broth, chicken, eight cups
Thyme, .5 teaspoon
Celery, two stalks dice
Carrots, three, peeled and diced
Onion, one, diced
Garlic, four cloves, minced

Salt and black pepper, .5 teaspoon each

Chicken thighs, one pound, boneless, skinless, cut in chunks

Olive oil, two tablespoons, divided

Set large pot over heat and warm one tablespoon olive oil. Add chicken thigh meat with salt and pepper and cook five minutes. Add rest of oil and celery, carrots, onion, garlic, and thyme and cook five minutes stirring often. Pour in broth and bay leaves and boil. Lower heat and stir in beans, simmer fifteen minutes. Add dill, parsley, lemon juice, and spinach and cook five minutes and serve.

Nutrition info: Calories 241, 9 grams fat, 1599 milligrams sodium, 18 grams carbohydrates, 4 grams fiber, 1 gram sugar, 19 grams protein.

Greek Spring Soup

Prep ten minutes/cook twenty-five minutes/serves four to six

Ingredients:

   Chives, fresh minced for garnish
   Salt and pepper, .25 teaspoon each
Dill, fresh, chop .5 cup
Carrots, one cup, diced
Asparagus, one cup, chopped
Lemon juice, two tablespoons
Egg, one
Arborio rice, .3 cup
Bay leaf, one
Onion, one small, diced
Olive oil, two tablespoons
Chicken, 1.5 cups cooked, diced
Broth, chicken, six cups

Use a large pot to cook the onions five minutes. Pour in .25 cup of dill, bay leaf, and chicken broth and boil.

Mix in the rice and lower heat; simmer ten minutes. Put in asparagus and carrots and simmer ten more minutes. Continue simmering while adding chicken, stir well. In a bowl blend two tablespoons of water with the lemon juice and the egg. Pour a half cup of the hot soup into the egg, stirring well, then add the egg mixture to the soup, stirring constantly. Remove the bay leaf when the soup has thickened. Garnish with the fresh dill.

Nutrition info: Calories 341, 9.7 grams fat, 934 milligrams sodium, 30 grams carbs, .4 grams fiber, 1.3 grams sugar, 31 grams protein.

Moroccan Lentil Soup

Prep twenty minutes/cook forty-five minutes/serves six to eight

Ingredients:

Salt and pepper, .25 teaspoon each
Chicken broth, low salt, eight cups
Whole tomatoes, canned, twenty-eight ounce, mashed with juice
Chickpeas, one fifteen-ounce can, drained and rinsed
Red lentils, dry, 1.25 cups, rinsed
Sweet paprika, two teaspoons
Cinnamon, one teaspoon
Turmeric, one teaspoon
Ginger, minced, two tablespoons
Cilantro, .5 cup, chopped
Parsley, .3 cup, chopped
Celery, two stalks, finely chopped
Onion, yellow, one, finely chopped
Olive oil, two tablespoons

Cook ginger, garlic, carrots, celery, and onion in hot oil for ten minutes, stirring often. Stir in salt, pepper, paprika, cinnamon, and turmeric, cooking five minutes to mix well. Pour in broth and tomatoes and mix well. Lower heat to simmer and stir in the parsley, cilantro, chickpeas, and lentils. Simmer soup for thirty minutes.

Nutrition info two cups: Calories 238, 7.3 grams fat, 86.2 milligrams sodium, 6.2 grams fiber, 32 grams carbs, 2.3 grams sugar, 14 grams protein.

Roasted Red Pepper and Tomato Soup

Prep ten minutes/cook forty-five minutes/serves four

Ingredients:

Cayenne pepper, .25 teaspoon
Paprika, ground, .25 teaspoon
Italian seasoning, .25 teaspoon
Parsley, fresh, chop, .25 cup
Tomato paste, two tablespoons
Broth, vegetable, two cups
Black pepper, .25 teaspoon
Salt, .25 teaspoon
Olive oil, two tablespoons
Garlic, two cloves, peeled and halved
Onion, one medium, cut in quarters
Tomato, three, cored and halved
Red bell peppers, two, seeded and cut in half

Heat oven to 400. In a bowl toss the garlic, onion, tomatoes, and red pepper with the salt, pepper, and oil. Place veggies on a baking pan and bake for forty-five minutes. Heat the broth and add the roasted vegetables to the broth, then puree the soup and put it back in the pot just until warm, stirring well.

Nutrition info one cup: Calories 150, 3.2 grams fat, 587.5 milligrams sodium, 14.4 grams carbs, 3.3 grams fiber, 1.6 grams sugar, 3.3 grams protein.

Mediterranean White Bean Soup

Prep fifteen minutes/cook eight hours/serves six

Ingredients:

Salt, one teaspoon
Thyme, dried, one teaspoon
Sage, dried, .5 teaspoon
Rosemary, dried, .5 teaspoon
Basil, dried, .5 teaspoon
Navy beans, two cups, dried
Broth, low sodium vegetables, six cups
Garlic, four cloves, minced
Onion, one medium, chopped
Celery, one cup, chopped
Carrots, one cup, chopped

Mix all ingredients in a crockpot. Cook low temperature for eight hours.

Nutrition info: Calories 183, 9.3 grams fat, 504 milligrams sodium, 21.8 grams carbs, 3.7 grams fiber, 1.1 grams sugar, 4.5 grams protein.

Minestrone

Prep twenty minutes/cook one hour/serves eight

Ingredients:

Cheese, Parmesan or Romano, .25 cup, shredded
Spinach, fresh, baby, four cups
Pasta shells, small, .75 cup
Black pepper, .5 teaspoon
Salt, one teaspoon
Thyme, .25 teaspoon
Basil, .5 teaspoon
Oregano, 1.5 teaspoon
Water, two cups
Broth, vegetables, four cups
Diced tomatoes, fire roasted, one fourteen- to fifteen-ounce can
Kidney beans, red, two fifteen-ounce cans, rinsed and drained
Cannellini beans, two fifteen ounce cans, rinsed and drained
Olive oil, three tablespoons

Celery, .5 cup, sliced thin

Parsley, fresh minced, two tablespoons

Squash, one medium, yellow, thin slices

Zucchini, one medium, thin slices

Carrots, .5 cup, diced

Garlic, four cloves, minced

Onion, white, one small, minced

Cook celery, parsley, squash, zucchini, carrots, garlic, and onion in hot oil in large pot for five minutes stirring often. Pour in diced tomatoes, herbs, salt, pepper, kidney beans, cannellini beans, water, and broth and stir well to blend flavors. Boil mix, then lower heat and simmer for thirty minutes. Drop in the spinach and pasta and simmer thirty more minutes. Mix in the grated cheese and serve immediately.

Nutrition info: Calories 110, 1 gram fat, 810 milligrams sodium, 17 grams carbs, 4 grams fiber, 4 grams sugar, 5 grams protein.

Dairy-Free Zucchini Soup

Prep fifteen minutes/cook thirty minutes/serves eight

Ingredients:

Basil, fresh, .3 cup
Salt and pepper, .25 teaspoon each
Broth, chicken or vegetables, four cups
Garlic, four cloves, chopped
Olive oil, two tablespoons
Onion, one medium, diced
Zucchini, 2.5 pounds, sliced

Cook zucchini, garlic, and onion five minutes in hot oil, stirring often. Pour in broth and let simmer fifteen minutes. Mix in salt and pepper and then blend soup until creamy. Return to stove just until warm.

Nutrition info: Calories 79, 4.9 grams fat, 133 milligrams sodium, 8.8 grams carbs, 2.4 grams fiber, 3.2 grams sugar, 1.6 grams protein.

Tuscan Vegetables Pasta Soup

Prep ten minutes/cook twenty minutes/serves six to eight

Ingredients:

Parsley, fresh chopped for garnish
Salt, .5 teaspoon
Black pepper, one teaspoon
Basil, one tablespoon, chopped
Baby spinach, two cups chop
White beans, one fifteen-ounce can, rinsed and drained
Bow tie pasta, whole wheat, eight ounces
Tomato paste, two tablespoons
Broth, low-sodium vegetables, six cups
Diced tomatoes, one fifteen-ounce can
Zucchini, one medium, quartered and sliced
Celery, .5 cup, chopped
Carrot, .5 cup, chopped
Onion, yellow, one medium, diced

Garlic, four cloves, minced

Olive oil, two tablespoons

Cook garlic and onion in hot oil in large pot three minutes. Pour in zucchini, celery, and carrots and cook five minutes, stirring often. Mix in pepper, salt, and tomatoes and mix well, cooking two more minutes. Add in tomato paste and broth and bring to a boil. Lower to simmer and simmer ten minutes. Mix in basil, white beans, and spinach and blend well. Take from heat and let the mixture sit until the spinach wilts. Sprinkle on fresh parsley and serve.

Nutrition info: Calories 225, 5.2 grams fat, 256 milligrams sodium, 28.4 grams carbs, 5.8 grams fiber, 1.3 grams sugar, 17.7 grams protein.

Roasted Cauliflower and Cheddar Soup

Prep time five minutes/cook forty minutes/serves eight

Ingredients:

Cheddar cheese, 2.5 cups, shredded
Broth, chicken, five cups
Garlic, three tablespoons, minced
Onion, one-half medium, chopped
Garlic powder, one teaspoon
Sea salt, .5 teaspoon
Black pepper, one teaspoon
Cauliflower, one head, chopped
Olive oil, two tablespoons

Heat oven to 425. Mix chopped cauliflower with one tablespoon olive oil, garlic powder, salt and pepper to coat well. Bake on cookie sheet for thirty minutes. Use rest of the olive oil to cook onion in a large pot for five minutes. Place cooked cauliflower in the pot and stir for five minutes. Pour in broth and bring to a boil, then simmer for thirty minutes. Use a blender to puree the soup, then return to pot and stir in the cheese, mixing well.

Nutrition info: Calories 243, 8.3 grams carbs, 13.7 grams protein, 17 grams fat, 999.9 milligrams sodium, 2.3 grams fiber, 2.8 grams sugar.

Meatball Soup

Prep twenty minutes/cook twenty minutes/ serves three quarts

Ingredients:

MEATBALLS
Olive oil, three tablespoons
Black pepper, .5 teaspoon
Sea Salt, .5 teaspoon
Parsley, fresh, minced, two tablespoons
Bread crumbs, one cup
Egg, one
Parmesan cheese, fresh grated, .5 cup
Ground beef, lean, one pound

SOUP
Black peppercorns, .5 teaspoon, whole
Thyme, fresh, five sprigs
Bay leaves, two
Onion, one medium, diced

Tomato paste, three tablespoons

Broth, beef or chicken, two quarts

GARNISH if desired

Salt and pepper

Fresh parsley, chopped

Basil leaves, chopped

Freshly grated parmesan cheese

Mix all meatball ingredients except for the olive oil. Shape into tiny meatballs and fry in oil for ten minutes. Remove from the oil and set to the side. Put the diced onion in the oil and cook five minutes. Pour in the remaining soup ingredients and boil. Lower heat and simmer the soup for fifteen minutes. Add the meatballs back to the mix in the pot and simmer five more minutes. Serve with garnishes as desired.

Nutrition info one cup serving: Calories 277, 14 grams fat, 772 milligrams sodium, 26 grams carbs, 6 grams fiber, 0 grams sugar, 13 grams protein.

White Bean Soup with Sausage and Kale

Prep twenty minutes/cook twenty minutes/serves six

Ingredients:

Parmesan, shredded, .5 cup
Salt, .5 teaspoon
Black pepper, .5 teaspoon
Bay leaf, one
Rosemary, dried, one teaspoon
Cannellini beans, one twenty-eight ounce can, rinsed and drained
Broth, chicken, four cups
Kale, .5 pound, removed stems and chopped
Garlic, two cloves, chopped
Celery, one stalk, chopped
Carrot, one, peeled and chopped
Onion, one medium, peeled and chopped
Italian sausage, hot or sweet, one pound, diced
Olive oil, .25 cup

Brown sausage in hot oil in a large cooking pot for five minutes. Stir in garlic, celery, carrot, and onion and cook five minutes. Mix in bay leaf, rosemary, beans, and broth and boil. Lower heat and simmer for thirty minutes, stirring often.

Nutrition info: Calories 221, 8.6 grams fat, 621 milligrams sodium, 20.3 grams carbs, 4.7 grams fiber, 2.8 grams sugar, 15.9 grams protein.

Halibut Chowder

Prep twenty minutes/cook one hour ten minutes/serves eight

Ingredients:

Black pepper, .25 teaspoon
Thyme, dried, .25 teaspoon
Basil, dried, .5 teaspoon
Sea salt, .5 teaspoon
Parsley, fresh, chopped, two tablespoons
Whole peeled tomatoes, two sixteen ounce cans mashed with juice
Apple juice, .5 cup
Tomato juice, one cup
Olive oil, .25 cup
Garlic, three cloves, minced
Celery, three stalks, chopped
Onion, one medium, peeled and chopped
Red bell pepper, one, cleaned and chopped
Halibut steaks, cubed, 2.5 pounds

Cook garlic, onion, celery, and peppers in hot oil in large pot for five minutes. Mix in herbs, mashed tomatoes, apple juice, and tomato juice and stir well. Simmer this mix for thirty minutes. Drop halibut pieces into the soup while stirring. Add pepper and salt and simmer thirty minutes.

Nutrition info: Calories 262, 10.3 grams fat, 10.7 grams carbs, 31.2 grams protein, 400 milligrams sodium, 2.1 grams fiber.

Lamb Stew

Prep twenty-five minutes/cook one hour ten minutes/serves six

Ingredients:

Parsley, fresh chop, three tablespoons
Zucchini, two small, peeled and sliced
Red bell pepper, one, seeded and chopped
Green beans, fresh, two cups, trimmed
Potatoes, four, peeled and cubed
Bay leaf, one
Oregano, dried, one teaspoon
Tomatoes, peeled, chopped, four cups
Broth, chicken, .5 cup
Red wine, .5 cup
Garlic, five cloves, sliced thin
Sea salt, .5 teaspoon
Black pepper, one teaspoon
Lamb shoulder, boneless, 1.5 pounds, cubed
Olive oil, two tablespoons

Sprinkle pepper and salt on the lamb and cook with garlic in hot oil in large pot for five minutes. Mix in broth and red wine and boil. Lower heat and put in bay leaf, oregano, and tomatoes, stir well and simmer forty-five minutes. Bring back to almost boil and stir in zucchini, red pepper, green beans, and potatoes and cook twenty minutes, stirring often. Remove the bay leaf and sprinkle parsley on soup to serve.

Nutrition info: Calories 389, 16.7 grams fat, 238 milligrams sodium, 38 grams carbs, 7 grams fiber, 20.3 grams protein.

Pasta Faggioli

Prep ten minutes/cook one hour thirty minutes/serves eight

Ingredients:

Ditalini pasta, one pound, cooked by package directions
Parmesan cheese, grated, .3 cup
Navy beans, one fifteen-ounce can, drained and rinsed
Cannellini beans, one fifteen-ounce can, drained and rinsed
Salt, one teaspoon
Oregano, dried, 1.5 teaspoons
Basil, dried, 1.5 teaspoons
Parsley, one tablespoon
Water, 5.5 cups
Tomato sauce, one twenty-nine ounce can
Garlic, two cloves, minced
Onion, peeled and chunked
Olive oil, three tablespoons

Cook onion and garlic in a large pot in oil for five minutes. Lower heat and add Parmesan cheese, navy beans, cannellini beans, salt, oregano, basil, parsley, water, and tomato sauce, stir well and simmer one hour. Mix in cooked pasta and simmer five more minutes.

Nutrition info: Calories 403, 7.6 grams fat, 1223 milligrams sodium, 68 grams carbs, 8.4 grams fiber, 16.3 grams protein, 6 grams sugar.

Beef Barley Soup

Prep ten minutes/cook five hours/serves six

Ingredients:

Sea salt, .5 teaspoon
Black pepper, one teaspoon
Pearl barley, one cup, uncooked
Tomato sauce, one eight-ounce can
Onion, one half, chopped
Beef bouillon, two tablespoons, granulated
Water, five cups
Beef chuck roast, two pounds, cubed

Use a crockpot to cook barley, salt, pepper, tomato sauce, onion, bouillon, water, and beef for five hours on low.

Nutrition info: Calories 512, 27.8 grams fat, 884 milligrams sodium, 35.4 grams carbs, 5 grams fiber, 29.7 grams protein, 3 grams sugar.

Beef Stew

Prep thirty minutes/cook four hours thirty minutes/serves eight

Ingredients:

Tomato sauce, two cups
Broth, beef, one quart
Sage, dried, .5 teaspoon
Marjoram, dried, one teaspoon
Thyme, dried, one teaspoon
Basil, dried, one tablespoon
Red potatoes, 1.5 pounds, chunked
Tomatoes, four, chopped
Dry red wine, two cups
Garlic, two tablespoons minced
Mushrooms, button, one pound sliced
Carrots, four large chunked
Celery, chunked, two cups
Onions, two large diced
Top round, lean two pounds cubed
Olive oil, two tablespoons

Use a large skillet to brown beef in hot oil for five minutes. Take beef from oil and set to the side. Put carrots, celery, garlic, mushrooms, and onions in oil five minutes. Add wine to skillet and boil, then add tomatoes. Put beef back in the skillet with tomato sauce, broth, sage, marjoram, thyme, basil, and potatoes. Lower heat and simmer five hours.

Nutrition info: Calories 476, 10.2 grams fat, 500 milligrams sodium, 34.4 grams carbs, 7.2 grams fiber, 49.9 grams protein, 11 grams sugar.

Cabbage and Smoked Sausage Soup

Prep twenty minutes/cook one hour ten minutes/serves eight

Ingredients:

Thyme, crushed, .5 teaspoon
Bay leaf, one
Salt, .5 teaspoon
Bouillon, chicken, two cubes
Crushed tomatoes, one twenty-eight ounce can
Tomato sauce, one eight-ounce can
Red beans, one fifteen-ounce can with liquid
White rice, long grain, .3 cup, uncooked
Celery, three stalks, sliced
Carrots, three slices
Cabbage, one head, removed core and chopped
Water, three cups
Smoked sausage, one pound, sliced
Onion, one, chopped
Olive oil, one tablespoon

Cook onion in oil in large skillet five minutes. Stir water and sausage into the pot. Add in crushed tomatoes, tomato sauce, beans, rice, celery, carrots, and cabbage and mix well. Mix in thyme, bay leaf, salt, and bouillon. Boil one minute, then lower heat, simmer one hour.

Nutrition info: Calories 404, 20.6 grams fat, 1618 milligrams sodium, 37.4 grams carbs, 9.8 grams fiber, 20.3 grams protein, 10 grams sugar.

Creamy Chicken Tortellini Soup

Prep ten minutes/cook thirty minutes/serves four

Ingredients:

Black pepper, .25 teaspoon
Thyme, .25 teaspoon
Spinach, frozen, chopped, one ten-ounce pack, thawed and drained
Cream, two cups
Cream of chicken soup, two ten-ounce cans
Cheese tortellini, one nine-ounce package
Broth, chicken, one fifteen-ounce can
Chicken breast, .5 pound, cubed and cooked

Boil chicken broth and add tortellini. Lower heat and simmer ten minutes. Add black pepper, thyme, spinach, cream, soup, and chicken and cook ten minutes.

Nutrition info: Calories 529, 29 grams fat, 1645 milligrams sodium, 39.9 grams carbs, 4 grams fiber, 28.4 grams protein, 3 grams sugar.

Tuscan Fish Stew

Prep twenty-five minutes/cook twenty-five minutes/serves two

Ingredients:

Rosemary, fresh, .5 teaspoon, minced
Oregano, freshly chopped, .5 tablespoon
Basil, freshly chopped, .5 tablespoon
Parsley, freshly chopped, one tablespoon
Salt, .5 teaspoon
Shrimp, one pound, peeled and deveined
Halibut, twelve ounces, chunked
Red pepper flakes, .5 teaspoon
Garlic, four cloves, sliced
Green onions, .25 cup, sliced
Olive oil, four tablespoons, divided
Clam juice, one cup
cherry tomatoes, three cups, cut in half

Use a blender to puree clam juice and cherry tomatoes. Cook red pepper flakes, garlic, and green onions in three tablespoons of oil for five minutes. Pour in tomato mix, Simmer ten minutes. Mix in salt and fish and cook ten minutes. Stir in rosemary, oregano, basil, and parsley; mix well and serve.

Nutrition info: Calories 672, 34.1 grams fat, 922 milligrams sodium, 14.3 grams carbs, 3.3 grams fiber, 76.3 grams protein. 0 grams sugar.

Chapter 12: Dinner Recipes

Walnut Rosemary Salmon

Prep ten minutes/cook twenty minutes/serves four

Ingredients:

Spray oil
Dijon mustard, two teaspoons
Rosemary, chop fresh, one teaspoon
Panko breadcrumbs, three tablespoons
Salmon fillets, one pound fresh or frozen
Olive oil, one teaspoon
Walnuts, three tablespoons, finely chopped
Red pepper, crushed, .25 teaspoon
Salt, .25 teaspoon
Honey, .25 teaspoon
Lemon juice, one teaspoon
Lemon zest, .25 teaspoon
Garlic, one clove, minced

Heat oven to 425. Blend red pepper, salt, honey, rosemary, lemon juice, lemon zest, garlic and mustard in small bowl. In another small bowl mix the oil, walnuts, and panko crumbs. Lay salmon fillets on a cookie sheet. Coat each fillet with the mustard mix and cover with panko mix. Spray oil each fillet to set toppings. Bake fifteen minutes.

Nutrition info: Calories 222, 12 grams fat, 0 grams fiber, 4 grams carbs, 24 grams protein, 1 gram sugar, 256 milligrams sodium.

Baked Cod with Maple Mustard

Prep time thirty minutes/serves two to three

Ingredients

Cod, four ounces each fillet, two or three
Lemon juice, one teaspoon
Dijon mustard, three tablespoons
Poppy seed, one teaspoon
Onion, chopped, .25 cup
Salt and pepper, .25 teaspoon each
Mustard powder, .25 teaspoon
Maple syrup, two tablespoons (can be substituted by honey)
Garlic powder, .5 teaspoon
Oil, one tablespoon

Heat oven to 400 degrees. Mix salt, pepper, garlic poppy seed, mustard, maple syrup, oil, and mustard powder and set aside. Spread two tablespoons of mix on the top each fillet. Sprinkle chopped onion on fish. Bake for fifteen minutes. Drizzle with lemon juice before serving.

Nutrition info: Calories 211, 9.2 grams fat, 145.9 milligrams sodium, .4 grams carbs, 0 grams fiber, 0 grams sugar, 29 grams protein.

Chicken Thighs with Vegetables

Prep time one hour forty minutes/serves four

Ingredients:

Broth, chicken, two cups
Dijon mustard, two tablespoon
Chicken thighs, four, boneless, skinless
Oil, one tablespoon
Garlic, four cloves, diced
Cabbage, purple, one fourth
Onion, one yellow, diced
Carrots, four medium, peeled and chunked
Potato, russet, one large, peeled and chunked
Salt and pepper, .25 teaspoon each

Heat oven to 375 degrees. Use a large skillet to warm oil and place thighs in oil. Season with salt and pepper and cook seven minutes each side. Take chicken out of the pan and set to the side. Add garlic and bacon to the pan and cook for five minutes. Stir in the carrots, potato, and onion making sure to mix well with bacon fat. Use safe oven dish to put the mixture in and bake for twenty minutes. Add mustard, cabbage, and thighs to pan and bake an additional twenty minutes.

Nutrition info: Calories 348, 18 grams fat, 680 milligrams sodium, 30 grams carbs, 8 grams fiber, 7 grams sugar, 22 grams protein.

Almond Artichoke Chicken Breasts

Prep time one hour/serves four

Ingredients:

Chicken, breast, four, skinless, boneless
Oil, two tablespoons
Artichoke hearts, one can
Spinach, baby, one-half cup, chopped
Pepper, .5 teaspoon
Salt, .5 teaspoon
Parmesan cheese, grated, two tablespoons
Almonds, roasted, chopped, two tablespoons

Combine spinach, almonds, Parmesan, half of the pepper and the salt, and artichokes in a small bowl. Cut into the thickest part of each chicken breast, about two inches long. Stuff one-quarter of the mix in the bowl into each breast. Season tops of breasts with remaining salt and pepper. Fry the chicken breasts ten minutes each side.

Nutrition info: Calories 224, 5.6 grams fat, 377.9 milligrams sodium, 15.3 grams carbs, 7.5 grams fiber, 0 grams sugar, 29.9 grams protein.

Tuna Salad Nicoise

Prep time forty-five minutes/serves four

Ingredients:

SALAD
Tuna steaks, two eight ounces each
  Hard-boiled eggs, two, sliced
French style green beans, four ounces
Oil, one tablespoon
Bibb lettuce, one large head
Red potato wedges, twelve ounces
Red onion, thin sliced, .5 cup
Grape tomatoes, one cup
Basil leaves, .5 cup
Black olives, pitted, .25 cup
Salt and pepper, .25 teaspoon each

DRESSING
Lemon juice, two tablespoons
Water, one tablespoon
Oil, three tablespoons

Garlic, one clove, minced

Salt and pepper, .25 teaspoon each

Sugar, .5 teaspoon

Use a small bowl to mix all the dressing ingredients, then refrigerate. Cook the green beans two minutes in water and then drain well. Using a large skillet over medium heat warm one tablespoon oil and cook the potatoes five minutes each side, stirring well and often. Arrange Bibb lettuce leaves and basil evenly on four plates. Divide the potatoes, onions, green beans, olives eggs, and tomatoes evenly over four plates. Add the leftover oil to the skillet and cook the tuna, three minutes on each side. Season with salt and pepper. Cut tuna across the grain and divide evenly over plates. Serve with the chilled dressing.

Nutrition info: Calories 413, 9.4 grams fat, 386.8 milligrams sodium, 20.8 grams carbs, 4.8 grams fiber, 1.5 grams sugar, 57.5 grams protein.

Mustard Crusted Salmon Fillets with Roast Cauliflower

Prep time one hour/serves four

Ingredients:

Salmon fillets, four six-ounce each
Cauliflower, six cups florets
Lemon juice, two teaspoons
Fresh dill, chopped, two teaspoons
Honey, one tablespoon
Dijon mustard, three tablespoons
Salt, .25 teaspoon
Pepper, one teaspoon
Oil, two tablespoons

Heat oven to 400 degrees. Bake the florets on baking pan for twenty-five minutes. In a small bowl mix well the juice, honey, mustard, and dill. Lay salmon fillets skin side down on a foil covered baking sheet and season with salt and pepper. Cover fillets with the mustard mix. Bake an additional fifteen minutes.

Nutrition info: Calories 305, 11.6 grams fat, 2024 milligrams sodium, 10.2 grams carbs, .3 grams fiber, .3 grams sugar, 36.5 grams protein.

Roasted Whole Chicken with Lemons and Fennel

Prep time one hour fifteen minutes/serves four

Ingredients:

Lemons, two whole, cut in wedges
Chicken, one whole six to seven pounds
Salt, .5 teaspoon
Pepper, one teaspoon
Oil, one tablespoon
Fennel, two whole bulbs, cut in slices

Heat oven to 400 degrees. Cover large cookie sheet with foil and set the whole chicken in the center. In a small bowl toss the fennel and the lemons with oil and season with salt and pepper. Scatter on baking sheet around chicken. Bake for one hour or until chicken juices run clear.

Nutrition info: Calories 387, 24 grams fat, 5 grams fiber, 12 grams carbs, 31 grams proteins, 5 grams sugar, 501 milligrams sodium.

Caprese Stuffed Portobello Mushrooms

Prep twenty five minutes/cook fifteen minutes/serves four

Ingredients:

Balsamic vinegar, two teaspoons
Fresh basil, .5 cup, thin slices
Mozzarella pearls, fresh, .5 cup, drained and pat dry
Cherry tomatoes, one cup, cut in half
Portobello mushrooms, four, removed stems and gills*
Black pepper, .25 teaspoon
Salt, .25 teaspoon
Garlic, one clove, minced
Olive oil, three tablespoons, divided

Heat oven to 400. Blend well garlic, two tablespoons of oil, and half of the salt and the pepper. Coat mushrooms well with oil mix using a food brush. Set mushroom on a cookie sheet and bake ten minutes. While the mushrooms are baking mix the basil, mozzarella, tomatoes, and the other half of the salt and pepper in a bowl. After the mushrooms have baked fill them with the tomato cheese mix. Bake fifteen more minutes until cheese is melted. Use vinegar to garnish mushrooms before serving.

Prepare the mushroom caps by gently twisting off the stems from the Portobello's. Using a spoon scrape off the gills from the underneath side of the caps. The indention should be smooth when you are done. You may also purchase Portobello caps if you prefer.

Nutrition info one mushroom: Calories 186, 16 grams fat, 2 grams fiber, 6 grams carbs, 6 grams protein, 4 grams sugar, 313 milligrams sodium.

Vegetarian Salad Nachos

Prep fifteen minutes/serves six

Ingredients:

Oregano, fresh, one tablespoon, minced
Red onion, two tablespoons, minced
Black olives, two tablespoons, chopped
Feta cheese, .25 cup, crumbled
Grape tomatoes, .5 cup, cut in quarters
Romaine lettuce, one cup, chopped
Pita chips, three cups whole grain
Black pepper, .25 teaspoon
Lemon juice, one tablespoon
Olive oil, two tablespoons
Hummus, .3 cup, prepared

Blend together pepper, lemon juice, oil, and hummus in a bowl. Spread a layer of pita chips on a platter. Use a spoon to dribble three-fourths of the hummus mix over the chips. Garnish the chips with red onion, olives, feta cheese, tomatoes, and lettuce. Spoon remainder of hummus decoratively in the middle and garnish with oregano.

Nutrition info: Calories 159, 10 grams fat, 2 grams fiber, 13 grams carbs, 4 grams proteins, 2 grams sugar, 270 milligrams sodium.

Chicken with Roasted Vegetables and Lemon Vinaigrette

Prep thirty minutes/cook forty-five minutes/serves four

Ingredients:

Balsamic vinegar, two tablespoons
Black olives, ten large, pitted
Cherry tomatoes, red or yellow, one cup
Cannellini beans, one fifteen- to sixteen-ounce can, drained and rinsed
Asparagus spears, one pound, fresh, trimmed and cut in two inch pieces
Olive oil, one tablespoon
Garlic, two cloves, minced
Bell pepper, red or green, one, cleaned and chopped
Red onion, one, peeled and sliced
Mushrooms, fresh, sliced, one cup
Chicken, thighs or breasts, 1.5 pounds skinless, boneless

Black pepper, .5 teaspoon

Salt, .25 teaspoon

Rosemary, freshly chopped, one teaspoon

Basil, freshly chopped, one tablespoon

Oregano, freshly chopped, one tablespoon

Parsley, freshly chopped, two tablespoon

Heat oven to 425. Spray oil two eleven by seventeen (or comparable size) baking dishes and set to the side. Mix pepper, salt, rosemary, basil, oregano, and parsley in a bowl. Lay chicken in one of the baking dishes. Use half of the herb mix to sprinkle over the chicken. Use a large bowl to toss together oil, garlic, bell pepper, onion, and mushroom. Pour this mix in the other baking dish. Bake both dishes together for thirty minutes. If the chicken is done cooking cover the pan to keep it warm and set to the side. Mix the balsamic vinegar, olives, tomatoes, beans, and asparagus with the roasted vegetables and sprinkle with remaining herb mix and combine well. Bake fifteen more minutes.

Nutrition info two cup serving: Calories 360, 12 grams fat, 9 grams fiber, 27 grams carbs, 43 grams protein, 6 grams sugar, 524 milligrams sodium.

Chicken with Balsamic Tomato Sauce

Prep thirty-five minutes/serves four

Ingredients:

Butter, one tablespoon
Fennel seeds, toasted, one tablespoon
Garlic, minced, one tablespoon
Broth, chicken, low sodium, one cup
Balsamic vinegar, .25 cup
Shallots, sliced, two tablespoons
Cherry tomatoes, .5 cup, cut in half
Olive oil, three tablespoons, divided
Whole wheat flour, .25 cup
Salt, .25 teaspoon
Chicken breast, two eight ounces, boneless, skinless

Cut both chicken breasts in half, lengthwise, then pound with meat mallet until each breast is about one-fourth-inch thick. Dash on salt and pepper very lightly. Cover breasts with flour (throw away rest of the flour). Fry the chicken in the oil in a large skillet for three or four minutes on each side until the chicken is brown. Lay chicken on a plate, cover with aluminum foil, and set to the side. Pour in the rest of the oil and put the shallot, tomatoes, and vinegar in the skillet and cook one minute. Add the leftover pepper and salt along with the fennel seeds, garlic, and the broth. Cook this mixture for five to nine minutes stirring in the butter as it cooks. Cover the chicken pieces with the sauce to serve.

Nutrition info: Calories 294, 17 grams fat, 1 gram fiber, 9 grams carbs, 25 grams proteins, 3 grams sugar, 371 milligrams sodium.

White Fish with Lemon Orzo

Prep fifteen minutes/cook fifteen minutes/serves four

Ingredients:

SAUCE

Sea salt, .25 teaspoon

Black pepper, .5 teaspoon

Crushed tomatoes, one fifteen-ounce can

Black olives, sliced, two tablespoons

Capers, two tablespoons, rinsed and drained

Oregano, fresh chop, one tablespoon

Anise seed, dried, one teaspoon

Crushed red pepper, .5 teaspoon

Shallots, two, minced

Garlic, minced, one teaspoon

Olive oil, one tablespoon

FISH

Parsley for garnish

Feta cheese, one ounce, crumbled

White fish fillets, four six-ounce, rinsed and dried

LEMONY ORZO

Broth, chicken or vegetables, three cups

Shallot, one, minced

Olive oil, one teaspoon

Orzo paste, one cup

Lemon juice, two tablespoons

Lemon zest, two tablespoons

Sea salt, .5 teaspoon

Black pepper, one teaspoon

Heat oven to 400.

TO MAKE SAUCE: Cook crushed red pepper, shallots, and garlic in olive oil using medium heat for five minutes. Stir in the oregano, tomatoes, capers, and anise seed and simmer five minutes. Take the pan of sauce off the heat and set to the side.

TO MAKE FISH: Spray oil a nine by thirteen baking dish and scoop two thirds (roughly) of the tomato sauce mixture into the dish. Lay the fish on top of the sauce. Pour the rest of the sauce directly down the center of the fish. Bake the fish ten minutes. Then sprinkle the feta cheese over the fish and bake five more minutes.

TO MAKE LEMONY ORZO: Before placing the fish in the oven, start the broth to boiling. Pour the olive oil in a skillet and cook the shallots five minutes. Stir in the lemon juice, lemon zest, and orzo. Then start adding the hot broth to the skillet using a large spoon, one spoon at a time. Let the orzo absorb the liquid before adding the next spoonful. Stop adding broth when the orzo is al dente.

TO SERVE: Carefully use a spatula to transfer fish fillet to a plate. Place a scoop of the Lemony Orzo beside each fillet. Sprinkle chopped parsley over all.

Nutrition info: Calories 402, 21 grams fat, 27 grams carbs, 31 grams protein

Hasselback Caprese Chicken

Prep twenty five minutes/cook twenty-five minutes/serves four

Ingredients:

Olive oil, two tablespoons
Broccoli florets, eight cups
Pesto, prepared, .25 cup
Mozzarella, fresh, three ounces, halved and sliced
Tomato, one medium, sliced
Black pepper, .25 teaspoon and .25 teaspoon
Salt, .25 teaspoon and .25 teaspoon
Chicken breast, two, boneless, skinless

Heat oven to 375. Spray oil a cookie sheet. Cut slices across each chicken breast about one-half inch apart from one end to the other. Use one each of the salt and pepper to sprinkle on the chicken. Alternately fill the cut places with cheese and tomato. Coat with pesto. Lay the chicken down one side of the cookie sheet. Put the rest of the salt and pepper with the oil and the broccoli in a bowl and toss well until the broccoli is well coated. Put the broccoli on the empty side of the cookie sheet, adding in any tomatoes that are leftover. Bake for thirty minutes.

Nutrition info: Calories 355, 19 grams fat, 4 grams fiber, 10 grams carbs, 38 grams protein, 3 grams sugar, 634 milligrams sodium.

Poached Fish in Basil Tomato Sauce

Prep fifteen minutes/cook thirty minutes/serves four

Ingredients:

Basil leaves, fresh, .25 cup fine chop + more for garnish if desired
Black pepper, .5 teaspoon
Sea salt, .25 teaspoon
Broth, .75 cup
Garlic, two cloves, peeled and sliced thin
Cherry tomatoes, two cups, cut in half
White fish fillets, four six-ounce fresh or thawed frozen

Cook garlic, salt, pepper, and tomatoes in hot oil for five minutes. Pour in the broth and add the chopped basil and the fish fillets. Cover the skillet and cook at a simmer for twenty-five minutes. Serve the cooked fish with couscous or rice as is desired.

Nutrition info: Calories 180, 1.9 grams fat, 454 milligrams sodium, 5.3 grams carbs, 1.4 grams fiber, 3 grams sugar, 33.8 grams protein.

Mediterranean Pasta

Prep five minutes/cook fifteen minutes/serves four to six

Ingredients:

Parsley, fresh chopped, .25 cup
Parmesan cheese, fresh grated, .25 cup
Lemon juice, .25 cup
Red pepper flakes, .5 teaspoon
Black pepper, .5 teaspoon
Olive oil, three tablespoons
Black olives, six ounces whole, pitted
Artichoke hearts, one fourteen-ounce can, quartered
Grape tomatoes, two cups
Garlic, four cloves
Angel hair pasta, whole wheat, six ounces
Sea salt, one tablespoon + one teaspoon

Cook the pasta per the package directions with one tablespoon salt until al dente. Drain the pasta but save half the sauce. During the time the pasta is cooking get the veggies ready by slicing the olives, chopping the artichokes, cut the cherry tomatoes in half, and mince the garlic. Use a large skillet to cook the red pepper flakes, pepper, one teaspoon salt, garlic, and tomatoes for three to five minutes. Drop the drained pasta into the skillet and stir rapidly. Mix in the lemon juice, olives, and artichokes. If this pasta mix seems dry use a bit of the saved pasta water to loosen it. When fully mixed take the skillet from the heat and garnish with the parsley and the Parmesan.

Nutrition info: Calories 267, 13 grams fat, 27 grams carbs, 3 grams fiber, 4 grams sugar, 18 grams protein.

Chicken Quinoa Bowl

Prep thirty minutes/serves four

Ingredients:

Parsley, fine chop, two tablespoons
Feta cheese, .25 cup crumbled
Cucumber, diced, one cup
Red onion, finely chopped, .25 cup
Black olives, pitted and chopped, .25 cup
Quinoa, two cups, cooked
Red pepper, crushed, .25 teaspoon
Cumin, ground, .25 teaspoon
Paprika, one teaspoon
Garlic, one clove, crushed
Olive oil, four tablespoons, divided
Almonds, slivered, .25 cup
Roasted red peppers, one seven-ounce jar, rinsed
black pepper, .25 teaspoon
Salt, .25 teaspoon
Chicken breast, one pound, boneless, skinless

Turn on oven broiler to high and set rack about eight inches below. Cover a cookie sheet with aluminum foil and put the breasts on it, using half the salt and pepper to season. Turn once while broiling eighteen to twenty minutes until meat thermometer says 165 degrees in thick part of the breast. Place the chicken breast on a plate and shred or slice very thin.

While the chicken is broiling puree the red pepper, cumin, paprika, garlic, almonds, and roasted peppers with two tablespoons of the oil until smooth. Use a bowl to mix the red onion, olives, quinoa, and the other two tablespoons of oil very well.

Spoon the quinoa mix into four bowls evenly divided. Top with the chicken and the cucumber. Drizzle on the red pepper sauce. Garnish with parsley and feta.

Nutrition info: Calories 519, 27 grams fat, 4 grams fiber, 31 grams carbs, 34 grams proteins, 3 grams sugar, 684 milligrams sodium.

Mediterranean Fish en Papillote

Prep five minutes/cook twelve minutes/serves two

Ingredients:

DRY RUB

Black pepper, .25 teaspoon

Salt, .25 teaspoon

Nutmeg, .25 teaspoon

Cinnamon, .25 teaspoon

Sage, ground, .25 teaspoon

Onion powder, .25 teaspoon

Thyme, dried, one teaspoon

Garlic powder, one teaspoon

FISH

Olive oil, two tablespoons

Red onion, three slices

Capers, drained, two teaspoons

Black olives, .5 cup

Artichokes, one cup

White fish fillets, two six ounces, skinless, boneless

Heat oven to 425. Blend the ingredients for the dry rub well in a small bowl. Tear off two sheets of aluminum foil just over one foot wide (about fourteen inches). Lay one fillet on each foil sheet. Sprinkle each fillet with one to two teaspoons of the rub mix (extra can be saved for another use). Place the capers, onions, artichokes, and olives over the fish fillets. Dribble olive oil over the veggies. Wrap the foil packets closed by pulling all sides to the top of the fish and rolling the pouch closed. Bake fifteen minutes on a cookie sheet.

Nutrition info: Calories 180, 63 grams fat, 101.2 milligrams sodium, 10.3 grams carbs, 4 grams fiber, 2.6 grams sugar, 22.4 grams protein.

Feta Chicken Pasta

Prep five minutes/cook thirty minutes/serves four to six

Ingredients:

Basil, fresh, finely chopped for garnish
Feta cheese, four ounces, divided
Whole wheat fettuccine, one pound
Water, two cups
Diced tomatoes, two fourteen ounce cans with spices
Black pepper, .25 teaspoon
Salt, one teaspoon, divided
Chicken breast, 1.5 pounds, boneless, skinless, chunked
Olive oil, two tablespoons

Cook chicken breast chunks in hot oil in large pot for ten minutes, stirring often to cook all sides of chicken. Sprinkle on half the salt and the pepper while stirring. Pour in the water and the diced tomatoes. Break pasta in half and stir in, cooking for ten minutes. Stir in three-fourths of the feta cheese. Cook for five more minutes. Garnish with fresh basil and the rest of the feta cheese.

Nutrition info: Calories 390, 11 grams fat, 531 milligrams sodium, 56 grams carbs, 6 grams fiber, 6 grams sugar, 19 grams protein.

Chicken Parmesan Pasta

Prep forty-five minutes/serves four

Ingredients:

Basil, fresh, chopped, .25 cup
Parmesan cheese, shredded, .25 cup
Mozzarella cheese, shredded, .5 cup
Whole wheat penne, eight ounces
Tomatoes, crushed, 1.5 cups
Broth, chicken, low sodium, three cups
Salt, .25 teaspoon
Italian seasoning, one teaspoon
Chicken breast, one pound, boneless, skinless, cut into cubes
garlic, minced, one tablespoon + one teaspoon
Panko breadcrumbs, whole wheat, .25 cup
Olive oil, two tablespoons

Brown garlic, salt, Italian seasoning, chicken, and panko in oil in a large skillet five minutes. Pour in the tomatoes and the broth and stir in the pasta. Boil and cook fifteen to twenty minutes until pasta is soft. Sprinkle with mozzarella cheese, basil, and Parmesan. Let sit five minutes before serving.

Nutrition info 1.5 cup serving: Calories 538, 17 grams fat, 7 grams fiber, 56 grams carbs, 41 grams protein, 7 grams sugar, 612 milligrams sodium.

Tuna Casserole

Prep twenty minutes/cook thirty minutes/serves twelve

Ingredients:

Sharp cheddar, shredded, three cups
Greek yogurt, plain, .5 cup
Milk, two cups
Sweet peas, frozen, .5 cup
Corn, whole kernel, frozen, .5 cup
Peas and carrots, frozen, one cup
Cream of Mushroom soup, one 10.5 ounce can
Tuna, twenty-four ounce can, canned in water
Whole grain pasta, one sixteen-ounce box, cooked to package directions

Heat oven to 375. Thoroughly mix two cups of the cheese with the yogurt, milk, all frozen vegetables, soup, tuna, and cooked noodles until well mixed. Spray oil nine by thirteen baking dish and spoon mix in. Bake for thirty minutes. Cover with the rest of the cheese and bake five more minutes.

Nutrition info one cup serving: Calories 232, 3.8 grams fat, 30 grams carbs, 22.7 grams protein, 4.8 grams fiber.

Creamy Tuscan Garlic Spaghetti

Prep five minutes/cook twenty minutes/serves four

Ingredients:

Black pepper, .25 teaspoon
Parmesan cheese, grated, .66 cup
Heavy cream, .5 cup
Olive oil, .25 cup
Water, four cups
Salt. One teaspoon
Italian seasoning, one tablespoon
Garlic, minced, one tablespoon
Baby spinach leaves, two cups
Onion, one medium, chopped
Roasted red peppers, one jar, chopped
Mushrooms, button, one cup, sliced
Spaghetti noodles, twelve ounces

Bring water, olive oil, salt, Italian seasoning, garlic, spinach, onion, red peppers, mushrooms, and spaghetti to a boil and cook fifteen minutes. Mix in the heavy cream and the parmesan and cook for five more minutes, stirring constantly. Stir in black pepper and serve.

Nutrition info: Calories 488, 35.8 grams fat, 607.6 milligrams sodium, 7.3 grams carbs, 1.2 grams fiber, 3.1 grams sugar, 33.8 grams protein.

Zucchini Lasagna Rolls

Prep forty five minutes/cook thirty minutes/serves four

Ingredients:

Almonds, chopped, .25 cup
Black pepper, .25 teaspoon
Parmesan cheese, grated, .25 cup
Ricotta cheese, part skim, 2.5 cups
Crushed red pepper, .25 teaspoon
Garlic, four cloves minced, divided Italian seasoning, one teaspoon
Crushed tomatoes, two cups
Salt, .25 teaspoon + .25 teaspoon
Olive oil, four tablespoons, divided
Zucchini, three large, trimmed

Heat oven to 425. Spray oil large cookie sheet. Cut slices from each zucchini down the length about one-quarter inch thick. Use three tablespoons of the oil to coat the strips and sprinkle on .25 teaspoon of salt.

Bake for twenty-five minutes until the strips are soft. Lower oven temp to 350. In a bowl mix the crushed red pepper, two teaspoons of the minced garlic, Italian seasoning, and the tomatoes and mix well. In another bowl mix well the black pepper, one teaspoon of the garlic, Parmesan, and ricotta cheese.

Pour the tomato mix into a greased nine by thirteen baking pan. Roll each strip of zucchini and place into tomato mix in pan. Spoon ricotta mix overall and bake thirty minutes. Garnish with the rest of the garlic and the chopped almonds.

Nutrition info per four rolls with sauce: Calories 324, 21 grams fat, 4 grams fiber, 19 grams carbs, 17 grams protein, 8 grams sugar, 447 milligrams sodium.

Spicy Salmon with Vegetable Quinoa

Prep ten minutes/cook twenty minutes/serves four

Ingredients:

QUINOA

Lemon zest, two tablespoons

Basil leaves, four, thin slices

red onion, .25 cup, diced

Cherry tomatoes, one cup, sliced in half

Cucumbers, .75 cup, diced

Salt, .5 teaspoon

Quinoa, one cup, cooked per package directions

SALMON

Parsley, freshly chopped, .25 cup

Lemon, one, cut into eight wedges

Salmon fillets, four five-ounce fillets

Paprika, .5 teaspoon

Cumin, one teaspoon

Black pepper, .25 teaspoon

Salt, .5 teaspoon

Heat oven to 400. Spray oil nine by thirteen baking dish. Place fish fillets in baking dish. Mix paprika, cumin, pepper, and salt in a small bowl and sprinkle on the fish. Lay the lemon wedges around the fish. Spoon the cooked quinoa around the fish. Use a medium bowl to toss together the lemon zest, basil, onions, tomatoes, and cucumber and pour over the fish and quinoa. Bake twenty minutes.

Nutrition info: Calories 222, 4 grams fat, 753 milligrams sodium, 16 grams carbs, 3 grams fiber, 2 grams sugar, 32 grams protein.

Shrimp Pasta with Lemon and Garlic

Prep ten minutes/cook twenty minutes/serves four

Ingredients:

Parsley, chopped, one tablespoon
Pasta any style, eight ounces
Lemon juice, two tablespoons
Lemon zest, one tablespoon
Red pepper flakes, .25 teaspoon
Garlic, one clove, minced
Grape tomatoes, one cup, halved
Zucchini, two cups, sliced thin
Olive oil, three tablespoons
Black pepper, .5 teaspoon
Salt, .5 teaspoon
Jumbo shrimp, one pound, deveined and peeled

Cook pasta per package directions. While the pasta is cooking cook zucchini with a dash of pepper and salt for five minutes. Mix in the tomatoes and cook three more minutes. Stir in the red pepper flakes, garlic, and shrimp and mix well. Cook for five minutes, stirring often until the shrimp is done. Stir shrimp mixture into drained cooked pasta and mix well.

Nutrition info: Calories 474, 15 grams fat, 481 milligrams sodium, 46 grams carbs, 3 grams fiber, 3 grams sugar, 37 grams protein.

Spinach and Feta Macaroni and Cheese

Prep five minutes/cook twenty minutes/serves four

Ingredients:

Parsley, chopped for garnish
Salt, .5 teaspoon
Black pepper, .5 teaspoon
Italian seasoning, .5 teaspoon
Milk, one cup
Broth, vegetables, one cup
Elbow macaroni, two cups
Mozzarella cheese, .25 cup, shredded
White cheddar cheese, .5 cup, cubed
feta cheese, .5 cup, crumbled
Baby spinach, fresh, eight to ten ounces
Tomatoes, two fresh, diced
Garlic, two cloves, minced
Onion, one, diced

Cook garlic and onions in hot oil for five minutes. Stir in seasonings, milk, broth, macaroni, cheeses, spinach, and tomatoes. Boil mix while stirring frequently, then turn down heat and simmer for fifteen minutes. Stir often, about every two to three minutes, or the mix will stick. Sprinkle with parsley and serve.

Nutrition info: Calories 544, 23 grams fat, 761 milligrams sodium, 60 grams carbs, 3 grams fiber, 6 grams sugar, 22 grams protein.

Apple Cherry Pork Medallions

Prep thirty minutes/serves four

Ingredients:

Brown rice, eight ounces, cooked
Cider vinegar, one tablespoon
Honey, one tablespoon
Cherries, dried tart, three tablespoons
Apple juice, unsweetened, .66 cup
Apple, one large, sliced
Olive oil, one tablespoon
Celery salt, .5 teaspoon
Thyme, dried, .25 teaspoon
Rosemary, dried, .25 teaspoon
Pork tenderloin, one pound

Slice tenderloin into twelve slices and sprinkle them with celery salt, thyme, and rosemary. Cook pork in hot oil three minutes each side; remove from skillet and set to the side. Add vinegar, honey, cherries, apple juice, and apple in skillet and mix well. Boil mix, then turn down the heat and simmer for five minutes. Put the pork back into the skillet and cook five more minutes. Serve pork mix with cooked rice.

Nutrition info for three ounces cooked pork and .3 cup of rice: Calories 349, 9 grams fat, 179 milligrams sodium, 37 grams carbs, 16 grams sugar, 4 grams fiber, 25 grams protein.

Black Bean and Sweet Potato Rice Bowl

Prep thirty minutes/serves four

Ingredients:

Sweet chili sauce, two tablespoons
Black beans, one fifteen-ounce can, drained and rinsed
Kale, fresh, four cups, chopped
Red onion, one, finely chopped
Olive oil, three tablespoons, divided
Water, 1.5 cups
Garlic salt, .25 teaspoon
Long grain rice, .75 cup, uncooked

Cook rice in water with garlic salt twenty minutes. While rice cooks put the sweet potato in oil in a skillet and cook eight minutes, stirring often. Mix in the kale, onion, and beans and cook five more minutes. Stir chili sauce into cooked rice and add to the potato mix; serve.

Nutrition info two cups: Calories 453, 8 grams fiber, 11 grams fat, 405 milligrams sodium, 10 grams protein, 74 grams carbs, 15 grams sugar.

Cod and Asparagus Bake

Prep thirty minutes/serves four

Ingredients:

Romano cheese, grated, .25 cup
Lemon zest, two teaspoons
Lemon juice, two tablespoons
Cherry tomatoes, one pint, cut in halves
Asparagus, one pound, trimmed
Cod fillets, four ounces each

Heat oven to 375. Spray oil nine by thirteen baking dish. Brush lemon juice on fish. Place cod in a baking dish and surround with tomatoes and asparagus. Sprinkle all ingredients with lemon zest and Romano cheese. Bake twenty minutes.

Nutrition info: Calories 141, 3 grams fat, 184 milligrams sodium, 6 grams carbs, 3 grams sugar, 2 grams fiber, 23 grams protein.

Beef and Blue Cheese Penne with Pesto

Prep thirty minutes/serves four

Ingredients:

Gorgonzola cheese, .25 cup, crumbled
Walnuts, .25 cup, chopped
Pesto, .prepared, .3 cup
Grape tomatoes, two cups, halved
Baby spinach, fresh, six cups, coarsely chopped
Black pepper, .25 teaspoon
Salt, .25 teaspoon
Beef tenderloin steaks, two, six ounces each
Penne pasta, whole wheat, two cups, cooked per package directions

While pasta is cooking broil the steaks five inches from heat seven minutes each side. After pasta is drained place in large bowl and stir in walnuts, pesto, tomatoes, and spinach; mix well. Slice steaks into quarter inch thick slices and toss with pasta. Garnish with cheese and serve.

Nutrition info: Calories 532, 22 grams fat, 434 milligrams sodium, 49 grams carbs, 3 grams sugar, 9 grams fiber, 35 grams protein.

Pepper Ricotta Primavera

Prep thirty minutes/serves six

Ingredients:

Fettucine, six ounces, cooked and drained
Basil, dried, .25 teaspoon
Oregano, dried, .25 teaspoon
Peas, frozen, one cup, thawed
Zucchini, one medium, sliced thin
Sweet Yellow pepper, one medium, cut julienne strips
Sweet red pepper, one medium, cut julienne
Red pepper flakes, crushed, .25 teaspoon
Garlic, one clove, minced
Olive oil, four teaspoons
Milk, .5 cup
Ricotta cheese, part skim, one cup

Blend milk and ricotta cheese and set to the side. Cook pepper flakes and garlic in hot oil two minutes. Stir in the sweet peppers, zucchini, peas, oregano, and basil and cook five minutes. Pour cheese mix over fettuccine; add vegetables from skillet and toss well.

Nutrition info one cup: Calories 229, 7 grams fat, 88 milligrams sodium, 31 grams carbs, 6 grams sugar, 4 grams fiber, 11 grams protein.

Chapter 13: Dessert Recipes

Italian Apple Olive Oil Cake

Prep twenty minutes/bake forty-five min

Ingredients:

Powdered sugar to dust pie with
Golden raisins, .66 cup, soak in warm water fifteen minutes to plump then drain
Eggs, two large
Olive oil, one cup
Sugar, one cup
Baking soda, one teaspoon
Baking powder, one teaspoon
Nutmeg, ground, .5 teaspoon
Cinnamon, ground, .5 teaspoon
Flour, all purpose, three cups
Orange juice, one cup, for soaking apples
Gala apples, two large, peeled and chopped finely

Heat oven to 350. Chop the apples and cover with orange juice to keep them from browning. Use a large bowl to sift baking soda, baking powder, nutmeg, cinnamon, and flour together. Set this bowl to the side. Blend together olive oil, sugar, and eggs for two minutes. Stir the wet and dry ingredients and mix until the two are just blended. The mixture will be somewhat thick but do not add any extra liquid to it. Drain the water off the raisins and the excess juice off the apples. Add both of these to the mix and stir well until all ingredients are well mixed. Spray oil a nine-inch cake dish and pour the batter into it. Smooth the top of the batter with the back of a spoon. Bake for forty-five minutes or until knife inserted in the center comes out clean. Dust with powdered sugar if desired.

Olive Oil Chocolate Chip Cookies

Prep twenty minutes/cook twelve min

Ingredients:

Chocolate chips, semisweet, two cups
Baking soda, .5 teaspoon
Flour, all purpose, two cups
Egg, one
Salt, one teaspoon
Brown sugar, light, .75 cup
Sugar, granulated, .75 cup
Vanilla, one tablespoon
Olive oil, one cup

Heat oven to 350. Spray oil two cookie sheets. Blend salt, both sugars, vanilla, olive oil, and egg until mixture is smooth. Stir in baking soda and flour. Gently mix in the chocolate chips. Form batter into balls, about two tablespoons of batter per ball, and place on the cookie sheets. Gently push the balls flat about the hallway. The cookies will bake for ten to twelve minutes. Cool the cookies for at least five minutes on the cookie sheet before moving to rack for cooling.

Mediterranean Brownies

Prep seven minutes/cook twenty-five minutes/makes twelve/calories per serving 150

Ingredients:

Walnuts, chopped, .3 cup
Salt, .25 teaspoon
Baking powder, .25 teaspoon
Cocoa powder, .3 cup
Flour, .5 cup
Eggs, two
Vanilla, one teaspoon
Sugar, .75 cup
Greek yogurt, .25 cup, low-fat
Olive oil, .25 cup

Heat oven to 350. Blend eggs, yogurt, vanilla, sugar, and olive oil until smooth. Use a separate bowl to mix together baking powder, salt, cocoa powder, and flour. Add the olive oil mix to the flour mix and blend well. Stir in the walnuts. Spray oil a nine-inch baking dish and spoon the batter into the dish. Bake for twenty-five minutes.

Greek Yogurt Chocolate Mousse

Prep five minutes/cook two hours/serves four/calories per serving 323

Ingredients:

Vanilla, .5 teaspoon
Honey, one tablespoon
Greek yogurt, two cups
Dark chocolate, 3.5 ounces
Milk, .75 cup

Chop the chocolate into fine pieces. Mix the chocolate shavings with the milk in a saucepan over low heat. Continue heating the milk until the chocolate melts completely, then blend in the vanilla and the honey. In a bowl mix the chocolate mix with the yogurt and blend together well. Pour into one large serving dish or several individual ones. Put mousse into the refrigerator for at least two hours before serving. This dessert can be garnished with fresh strawberry pieces or fresh raspberries if desired. This dessert will stay fresh in the refrigerator for two days.

Cinnamon Walnut Apple Cake

Prep twenty minutes/cook sixty minutes/yield twelve slices

Ingredients:

Sesame seeds, three tablespoons
Cinnamon, ground, 1.5 teaspoons
Raisons, .5 cup
Walnuts, chopped, .5 cup
Apples, four, peeled, halve cored, and sliced thinly
Vanilla, one teaspoon
Baking powder, two teaspoons
Wheat flour, 2.5 cups
Milk, one cup
Olive oil, one cup
Brown sugar, light, one cup plus two tablespoons
Eggs, four

Heat oven to 375. Cream together oil, sugar, and eggs. Stir in vanilla, baking powder, wheat flour, and milk and mix well, then beat mix for two minutes. Spray oil one nine inch square baking pan. Spoon half of the cake batter into the dish. Mix together the cinnamon, two tablespoons of brown sugar, raisins, walnuts, and apples and spoon this mix on top of cake batter in baking dish. Pour over the rest of the batter. Garnish top of batter with sesame seeds. Bake for forty-five to fifty minutes.

Peanut Butter Banana Greek Yogurt Bowl

Prep five minutes/serves four/calories 370 per serving

Ingredients:

Nutmeg, one teaspoon
Flaxseed meal, .25 cup
Creamy peanut butter, all natural, .25 cup
Bananas, two medium-sized, slice
Greek yogurt, vanilla flavor, four cups

Put yogurt in four bowls and place banana slices on top. Microwave the peanut butter thirty to forty seconds until soft and pour one tablespoon of peanut butter onto each bowl. Serve with a garnish of nutmeg and flaxseed meal.

Low-Fat Apple Cake

Prep time ten minutes/cook thirty-five minutes/serves eight/calories per slice 116

Ingredients:

Powdered sugar for garnish
Baking powder, three teaspoons
Milk, low fat, .25 cup + one tablespoon
Flour, all purpose, one cup
Salt, .25 teaspoon
Lemon zest, one tablespoon
Sugar, .3 cup
Eggs, two
Apples, 1.5 pound

Heat oven to 350. Spray oil a nine-inch baking dish. The apples should be cored, peeled, and then sliced very thinly. Cream together the salt, lemon zest, sugar, and eggs. Mix in the milk, baking powder, and flour and stir until well mixed. Pour two-thirds of the apple slices in the batter and fold the batter to mix the apples in.

Spoon the batter into the baking dish. Put the rest of the apple slices on top of the cake batter. Bake for thirty-five minutes. Garnish with powdered sugar for serving.

Popped Quinoa Crunch Bars

Prep five minutes/cook ten minutes/

Ingredients:

TOPPING
Peanut butter powder, 2.5 tablespoons
Water, two tablespoons

COOKIES
Vanilla, .5 teaspoon
Peanut butter powder, one tablespoon
Quinoa, one cup, dry
Chocolate bar, semi-sweet, sixteen ounces, chopped

Set a large pot with a heavy bottom over medium-high heat and allow the bottom to get hot for several minutes. Pour in one-fourth of the quinoa at a time and let it sit there, stirring occasionally. The quinoa will start popping, and when it does, begin to stir constantly and remove the quinoa from the pan when it is a golden color. Repeat this process with the other three batches of quinoa. Melt the chocolate in a double boiler.* Pour the melted chocolate into a bowl with the vanilla, peanut butter powder, and quinoa and mix until completely combined. Spray oil a cookie sheet and spoon this mix onto the sheet, flattening it until it is about one-quarter inch thick. The sides don't need to be perfectly shaped. While it is cooling mix the topping mix in a small bowl and use a spoon to dribble it over the quinoa mix. Swirl it into the chocolate with the tip of a knife. Cut when the mix is set.

*In place of a double boiler use two saucepans, one slightly smaller than the other one. Put two cups of water into the larger one and bring to a boil. Put the chocolate into the smaller one and set it in the large one as soon as the water begins boiling. Leave the heat turned on until the chocolate melts. Stir the chocolate frequently to prevent burning.

Chocolate Olive Oil Cake

Prep time ten minutes/cook thirty minutes

Ingredients:

Espresso powder, one teaspoon
Cocoa powder, four tablespoons
Salt, .25 teaspoons
Vanilla, one teaspoon
Eggs, five
Sugar, granulated, one cup
Olive oil, .5 cup
Dark chocolate, block, seven ounces, chopped finely

Heat oven to 350. Spray oil a nine inch round cake dish. Warm olive oil and chocolate, constantly stirring until chocolate is melted. Let cool five minutes. Mix in the vanilla, eggs, and sugar and keep mixing until batter is smooth. Stir in espresso powder, cocoa powder, and salt and mix well. Spoon the cake batter into the cake dish and bake for twenty-five to twenty-eight minutes. Leave the cake to cool in the dish for fifteen minutes before transferring to a plate or rack. This cake can be served with chocolate sprinkles, drizzles of chocolate or caramel syrup, a light dusting of powdered sugar, whipped cream, or ice cream

Maple Vanilla Baked Pears

Prep five minutes/cook twenty-five minutes/serves four

Ingredients:

Vanilla, one teaspoon
Cinnamon, ground, .25 teaspoon
Maple syrup, .5 cup
Anjou pears, four

Heat oven to 375. Spray oil cookie sheet. Cut each pear in half the long way. Then cut a tiny piece out of the outside of each half so they will sit still on the pan. Cover with ground cinnamon. Blend the vanilla and the maple syrup. Dribble all but two tablespoons over the pears. Bake for twenty-five minutes and dribble immediately with the rest of the vanilla maple mix.

Yogurt with Fresh Strawberries and Honey

Prep ten minutes/serves four

Ingredients:

Almonds, toasted and sliced, four tablespoons
Greek yogurt, plain, three cups
Honey, four teaspoons
Strawberries, fresh, one pint

Clean strawberries and slice, then set to the side. Spoon three-quarters of one cup of yogurt into four dessert dishes. Evenly divide the berries between the dishes. Garnish each dish with one teaspoon of the honey and one tablespoon of the almonds.

Tahini and Almond Cookies

Prep fifteen minutes/bake fifteen min

Ingredients:

Tahini paste, .75 cup + two tablespoons
Water, two tablespoons
Vanilla, one teaspoon
Sugar, .75 cup
Butter, .5 cup + three tablespoons, cut into cubes
Almond meal, .66 cup
Whole wheat flour, one cup + two tablespoons
White flour, one cup

Heat oven to 350. Spray oil two cookie sheets or cover with parchment paper. Cream together vanilla, sugar, water, tahini, and butter. Stir in almond meal and flours until dough is well mixed. Spoon tablespoons of the dough on to the cookie sheets, twelve per sheet. Bake for twelve to fourteen minutes or until the cookies are golden brown in color. Cool and serve.

Pear Cranberry Pie with Oatmeal Streusel

Prep fifteen minutes/bake one hour

Ingredients:

FILLING
Pie crust, one deep dish nine inch, unbaked
Cornstarch, 2.5 tablespoons
Light brown sugar, .5 cup packed
Cranberries, fresh, two cups
Pears, peeled and cubed, three cups

STREUSEL
Butter, one tablespoon cold, cut into bits
Nutmeg, ground, .25 teaspoon
Cinnamon, ground, .25 teaspoon
Brown sugar, light, .3 cup, packed
Oats, rolled, .75 cup

Heat oven to 350. Mix streusel by putting all the streusel ingredients into a bowl and mixing with two knives or a blender for pastry until mix is crumbly. Set this to the side. Mix corn starch, brown sugar, cranberries, and pears, mix well. Pour this mix into the pie shell and cover with the streusel mix. Bake for one hour and cool for one hour minimum before serving.

Fabulous Fig Bars

Prep thirty minutes/bake thirty min

Ingredients:

Oats, old fashioned rolled, 1.25 cup
Baking soda, .5 teaspoon
Flour, all purpose, 1.5 cups
Egg, one
Brown sugar, one cup, packed
Butter, .5 cup, room temp
Hot water, two tablespoons
Orange juice, .25 cup
Sugar, granulated, .3 cup
Walnuts, chopped, .5 cup
Dried figs, removed stems and chopped, sixteen ounces

Heat oven to 350. Spray oil nine by thirteen baking pan. Mix hot water, orange juice, sugar, walnuts, and figs and set to the side. Cream together egg, brown sugar, and butter until smooth. Mix baking soda and flour into egg mix, then mix in the oats. Place all but one cup of the dough into the baking pan and press with your fingers to cover the bottom. Spoon fig mix over the dough and use the back of a spoon to spread evenly. Drop small crumbles of the rest of the dough over the fig mix. Bake thirty minutes and cool completely before cutting into bars.

Strawberry Gelato

Prep thirty minutes/set twelve hours

Ingredients:

Strawberries, fresh, two pounds, cleaned and cut in quarters
Sugar, granulated, 1.25 cups
Heavy cream, three cups, divided
Cornstarch, two tablespoons

Blend together one-quarter cup of the cream with the cornstarch. Put the sugar with the rest of the cream in a pan and heat to simmer. Stir in cornstarch mixture. Increase heat until the mix boils, about ten minutes. Dump mix into a freezer safe bowl. Puree the strawberries and stir into the sugar mix. Cover and place bowl in a freezer for ten to twelve hours.

Chocolate Pistachio Biscotti

Prep one hour/bake one hour/makes three to four dozens

Ingredients:

Egg white, one, beaten
Pistachios, raw, 1.5 cups
Cinnamon, .5 teaspoons
Salt. .75 teaspoon
Baking powder, one teaspoon
Cocoa powder, unsweet, .5 cup
Flour, all purpose, 2.5 cups
Vanilla bean, one, scraped seeds
Eggs, two
Sugar, granulated, .75 cups
Butter, one stick, room temp

Heat oven to 350. Spray oil two cookie sheets. Cream together the vanilla seeds, eggs, sugar, and butter until smooth. Use another bowl to mix together the cinnamon, salt, baking powder, cocoa powder, and flour until well blended. Mix the two bowls together, adding the pistachios. Blend well. Place the dough on a lightly floured cutting board or counter and divide the dough into four evenly sized pieces. Roll the dough balls into log shapes about one and one-quarter inch thick. Place two log shapes on each cookie sheet and brush the tops with the beaten egg white. Bake the log shapes for twenty-five minutes and let cool ten minutes. Leave oven on. Cut the logs diagonally into slices about one-third of an inch thick. Lay the slices on the cookie sheets and bake for twenty minutes.

Almond Cake with Pears

Prep forty-five minutes/cook one hour thirty minutes/serves eight

Ingredients:

CAKE
Almond flour, 1.5 cups
Flour, all purpose, .25 cup
Orange zest, finely grated, one teaspoon
Salt
Sugar, one cup
Eggs, two large, beaten
Egg whites, six, beaten

PEARS
Powdered sugar for garnish
Bartlett pears, four, ripe firm, cut into half-inch wedges
Sugar, three tablespoons
Butter, three tablespoons

Heat oven to 350. Spray oil a ten-inch springform pan. Mix well the orange zest, a pinch of salt, all-purpose flour, almond flour, and one-half cup of the sugar, then add the eggs and mix well. In a separate bowl use a hand beater to whisk the egg whites with one salt pinch until they make soft peaks. Keep beating while pouring in the rest of the sugar and keep beating until the eggs form stiff peaks. Spoon the egg mixture into the flour mix gently until just mixed. Spoon the batter into the springform pan and bake for thirty minutes.

Leave the cake in the pan for fifteen minutes to cool and then put it on a rack to finish cooling. While the cake cools mix the butter with the sugar in a skillet and pour the pears in, stirring a few times. Simmer them in a covered pan for seven to ten minutes until the pears become tender. Cut the cooled cake with a serrated knife to cut the cake into two even layers. Use a large spoon to put the pear mix over the bottom layer and spread evenly, then return the top half of the cake and sprinkle the cake with powdered sugar to serve.

Greek Honey Cake

Prep thirty minutes/cook forty minutes/serves twelve

Ingredients:

Lemon juice, one teaspoon
Water, .75 cup
Honey, one cup
Sugar, white, one cup + .75 cup
Walnuts, chopped, one cup
Milk, .25 cup
Eggs, three
Butter, .75 cup
Orange zest, one teaspoon
Cinnamon, ground, .5 teaspoon
Salt. .25 teaspoon
Baking powder, 1.5 teaspoon
Flour, all purpose, one cup

Heat oven to 350. Spray oil one nine-inch square baking dish. Mix zest, cinnamon, salt, baking powder, and flour in a bowl and set to the side. Use another bowl cream together the butter, eggs, and .75 cup of sugar. Add the walnuts and the milk and mix well. Stir in the flour mixture until blended well. Spoon batter into baking dish and smooth top of batter with the back of the spoon. Bake for forty minutes. Let the cake cool for fifteen minutes before cutting. Serve with the honey syrup.

To make the honey syrup mix the water, one cup of sugar, and the honey in a pan and simmer for five minutes. Add in the lemon juice and let the mixture boil for two minutes.

Semolina Pudding

Prep fifteen minutes/cook thirty-five minutes/serves six

Ingredients:

Semolina flour, one cup
Butter, .5 cup
Cinnamon stick, one
Sugar, white, 1.5 cups
Milk, 15 cups
Water, one cup

Mix cinnamon, sugar, milk, and water in a pan and bring to a boil. Take the pan from the heat and take out the cinnamon stick. Use another pan to melt the butter, then add the semolina to the butter and mix well. Slowly add in the milk mix. Stir continuously until the mix has become thick. Pour mix into a gelatin type mold or into individual serving dishes. This can be served warm or cold. Garnish with honey or fresh fruit is desired.

Chapter 14: Snacks and Appetizers

Okay, let's face it; sometimes, we just need a little snack to tide us over until mealtime, or we're just not that hungry at mealtime and just want a little something, or maybe we're going to a house party and need to bring an appetizer and we want one that we know will fit into our personal dietary needs. So, here are a few snacks and appetizers (they can be either) to help keep the diet on track.

Smoked Salmon Feta Cheese Endive Bites

Ingredients:

Smoked salmon, one package
Feta Cheese, herbed, one package
Endive, three heads

Cut off the ends of the endive bunches and pull all the leaves off. Spread the leaves with feta cheese. Lay a slice of salmon on top of the cheese. Serve.

Fifteen-Minute Mediterranean Chickpea Salad

Ingredients:

Salt, .25 teaspoon
Black pepper, .5 teaspoon
Basil, fresh, finely chopped, three tablespoons
Parsley, fresh, finely chopped, .25 cup
Red wine vinegar, one tablespoon
Olive oil, two tablespoons
Lemon juice, two tablespoons
Feta cheese, plain or herbed, .25 cup
Black olives, sliced, .25 cup
Cucumber, finely chopped, .5 cup
Cherry tomatoes, one pint, cut in half
Chickpeas, one fifteen-ounce can, rinsed and drained

Place all these ingredients into a mixing bowl and mix together well.

Loaded Hummus

Ingredients:

HUMMUS

Salt, .5 teaspoon

Black pepper, one teaspoon

Water, four tablespoons

Cumin, .25 teaspoon

Paprika, .5 teaspoon

Lemon juice, one teaspoon

Garlic, one clove

Olive oil, three tablespoons

Tahini, two tablespoons

Chickpeas, one fifteen-ounce can, drained and rinsed

TOPPINGS

Cilantro, freshly chopped, two tablespoons

Sesame seeds, two tablespoons

Cucumber, chopped, .25 cup

Red onion, chopped, .25 cup

Cherry tomatoes, .25 cup

Chickpeas, .25 cup, crispy

Heat oven to 400. Put a quarter cup of chickpeas in the oven and bake for twenty-five minutes to make them crispy. Place all the hummus ingredients in a blender or a food processor and mix until smooth. Place the hummus onto a platter for serving and arrange the onion, cucumber, and tomatoes on top of the hummus. Garnish with the cilantro, sesame seeds, and crispy chickpeas. Arrange crackers or chunks of pita for dipping.

Baked Root Veggies with Parsley Buttermilk Dip

Ingredients:

PARSLEY BUTTERMILK DIP
Salt, .5 teaspoon
Honey, one teaspoon
Lemon zest, one teaspoon
Garlic, minced, two cloves
Parsley, minced, two tablespoons
Buttermilk, six tablespoons
Greek yogurt, low fat, one seven-ounce container

ROOT VEGGIE CHIPS
Cumin, ground, .5 teaspoon
Garlic powder, one teaspoon
Thyme, dried, .5 teaspoon
Olive oil, two tablespoons
Red beet, one medium
Golden beet, one medium
Parsnip, one large
Turnip, one medium

Heat oven to 400. Make the dip first. Mix the ingredients together, then cover and refrigerate until needed. Mix the salt, cumin, garlic powder, thyme, and oil in a bowl. Wash, dry, and peel the veggies and slice very thin. If you have a mandolin, it would be best for this. Using a pastry brush coat both sides of all veggies with the oil mix, then lay them on a rack placed on a cookie sheet. Bake chips for twenty minutes or a bit longer if needed until they are lightly browned and crispy. Serve warm or cooled with the dip.

Cucumber Bites with Salmon and Avocado

Ingredients:

Black pepper for garnish
Chives, chopped, for garnish
Smoked salmon, six ounces
Lime juice, .5 tablespoon
Avocado, one large, peeled and pit removed
Cucumber, one medium-sized

Peel cucumber if desired and slice it in slices about one-quarter inch thick, then lay the slices on a serving tray. Cream together the lime juice and avocado until smooth. Place a teaspoon of mashed avocado on each cucumber slice, then lay a slice of smoked salmon on top of the avocado. Use the chives and black pepper to garnish as desired.

Greek Yogurt Artichoke Spinach Dip

Ingredients:

Parmesan cheese, shredded, .3 cup
Mozzarella cheeses, shredded, .66 cup
Feta cheese, crumbled, one cup
Garlic, minced, two teaspoons
Greek yogurt, plain, 1.3 cups
Artichoke hearts, one fourteen-ounce, can drain and chop
Frozen spinach, thawed

Heat oven to 350. Spray oil an eight by eight baking dish. Squeeze excess liquid out of thawed spinach. Gently mix everything together. Pour mixture into baking dish and bake thirty minutes. Serve hot with veggies, crackers, or chips.

Roasted Chickpeas

Ingredients:

Black pepper, .5 teaspoon
Garlic powder, .5 teaspoon
Oregano, dried, one teaspoon
Salt, one teaspoon
Lemon juice, two teaspoons
Red wine vinegar, two teaspoons
Olive oil, two tablespoons
Chickpeas, two fifteen ounce cans, drained and rinsed

Heat oven to 425. Pour the chickpeas onto a cookie sheet. Bake the chickpeas for ten minutes, stir and bake for another ten minutes. Blend the rest of the ingredients very well in a mixing bowl. After the chickpeas have baked the second time pour them into the bowl of mix and toss them to coat well. Bake the chickpeas another ten minutes, cool and eat.

Loaded Eggplant Dip

Ingredients:

PUREE

Black pepper. .5 teaspoon

Salt, .25 teaspoon

Garlic, one clove minced

Lemon juice, two tablespoons

Olive oil, one tablespoon

Eggplant, one large

TOPPING

Lemon

Chives

Parsley

Olive oil

Pine nuts

Capers

Black olives

Heat oven to 400. Poke several holes carefully in the skin of the eggplant with a knife and rub lightly with olive oil. Bake the eggplant twenty minutes and let it cool to for twenty minutes. Remove the stem end and peel the whole eggplant. Mash the eggplant with pepper, salt, lemon juice, garlic, and olive oil until entire mixture is smooth. Refrigerate until ready to eat.

White Bean Artichoke Dip

Ingredients:

White beans, one fifteen-ounce can, drained and rinsed
Garlic, four cloves, peeled and smashed
Artichoke hearts, six-ounce can, marinated
Olive oil, two tablespoons
Basil, ground, two tablespoons
Cayenne pepper, .5 teaspoon
Lemon juice, two tablespoons

Puree in a blender the artichokes, garlic, and white beans (a food processor also works well for this). Then add the lemon juice, cayenne pepper, basil, and olive oil. Serve this dip with vegetable sticks or toasted pita bread chips.

Mediterranean Veggie Fritters

Ingredients:

Olive oil, three tablespoons for frying
Cornstarch, .25 cup
Egg, two
Beets, two medium, shredded
Lemon juice, .25 teaspoon
Parsley, chopped, two tablespoons
Black pepper, two teaspoons
Salt, one teaspoon
Coriander, ground, .25 teaspoon
Turmeric, .5 teaspoon
Cumin, two teaspoon
Carrots, grated, one cup
Scallions, thin slices, .25 cup
Garlic, two cloves, minced
Onions, two, minced

Cook garlic and onion in hot oil for three minutes, then place this in a mixing bowl. Add the cornstarch, lemon juice, parsley, spices, beets, carrots, and scallions. Mix well. In another bowl make a thick paste by beating the four and the eggs together. Add this paste to the veggie mix and stir together. Spoon the batter by tablespoons into hot oil and fry for three to five minutes on each side.

Tuna Stuffed Avocados

Ingredients:

Basil, fresh sliced for garnish
Black pepper, .5 teaspoon
Salt, .25 teaspoon
Black olives, minced, two tablespoons
Tomatoes, minced, two tablespoons
Pesto, 1.5 tablespoons
Albacore tuna, one can, drained
Avocado, one large, peeled

Cut the avocado in half long ways and remove the seed. Use a spoon to scrape out two tablespoons of flesh from each half. Place the scraped flesh in a mixing bowl. Add in the pesto and the tuna and mash this well and mix together. Next add in the olives, pepper, salt, and tomatoes and mix well. Spoon the mixture into the avocado and enjoy.

Greek Meatballs

Ingredients:

Olive oil, one tablespoon
Dill, ground, .25 teaspoon
Black pepper, .25 teaspoon
Garlic powder, .5 teaspoon
Salt, .5 teaspoon
Oregano, one teaspoon
Feta cheese, .5 cup
Red onion, grated, .25 onion
Turkey breast, ground, sixteen ounces

Turn on oven broiler and place rack five inches below. Mix all ingredients well. Scoop about one and one-half tablespoons of mix and form into meatball shape. Place meatballs on a spray-oiled cookie sheet. Broil ten minutes.

Tomato Parmesan Rosemary Palmiers

Ingredients:

Egg, one, beaten
Black pepper, .5 teaspoon
Rosemary, dried, one tablespoon
Parmesan cheese, grated, .25 cup
Tomatoes, finely chopped, .5 cup
Puff pastry, one sheet, ready rolled

Heat oven to 400. Put the sheet of puff pastry on a lightly floured counter or board and cover with the pepper, rosemary, parmesan, and tomatoes. Roll the long sides of the pastry and make them meet in the middle. Use a pastry brush to coat the two sides with beaten egg and then push the two sides together to make them stick to each other. Spray oil one cookie sheet. Carefully slice the roll into one inch thick slices and lay the slices on the cookie sheet. Bake fifteen minutes.

Baby Potatoes with Olive Pesto

Ingredients:

Sour cream, .5 cup
Garlic, two cloves, minced
Pine nuts, toasted, .25 cup
Onion, chopped, .5 cup
Green olives, pimiento stuffed, 1.5 cups
Salt, two teaspoons
Olive oil, six tablespoons, divided
Baby red potatoes, three pounds (about thirty-six)

Heat oven to 400. Wash and dry potatoes and put in a large bowl. Add two tablespoons of the oil and the salt and mix well. Spry oil a cookie sheet and put the potatoes on it; bake thirty minutes. While the potatoes are baking mix together the rest of the oil with the garlic, pine nuts, onion, and olives and blend until well chopped. After potatoes have cooled slice a thin slice off each bottom to allow them to sit upright. Slice two lines in the top of each potato making them cross in the middle and squeeze gently to open the cross. Use a teaspoon to fill each potato with the pesto mix and garnish with sour cream if desired.

Herb Cheese Bread

Ingredients:

Cheddar cheese, shredded, .75 cup
French bread, unsliced, one loaf
Red pepper flakes, .25 teaspoon
Salt, .25 teaspoon
Thyme, dried, .25 teaspoon
Oregano, dried, .25 teaspoon
Cumin, ground, .5 teaspoon
Butter, .3 cup, room temp
Garlic, two tablespoons, minced
Green onions, finely chopped, .25 cup

Heat oven to 400. Cut the loaf of bread in half from end to end. Cook garlic and onion in butter for three minutes, transfer to a bowl with the butter. Mix in all the seasonings. Use a knife to spread this mix over the inside halves of the bread. Wrap each bread half loosely in aluminum foil and bake, inside side up, for twenty-five minutes.

Chapter 15: Two Week Meal Plan

This is a suggestion for two weeks' worth of meals to help you get started on your healthy eating journey. Remember these are just suggestions, and you can feel free to substitute any of the recipes with any other recipes that might suit your personal tastes better. All of these recipes can be found in this book. Happy eating!

Day One
Breakfast   Kiwi Smoothie
Lunch   Eggplant and Millet Chickpea Stew
Dinner   Cabbage and Smoked Sausage Soup

Day Two

Breakfast   Spinach Mushroom Omelet

Lunch   Cucumber Tomato Toast

Dinner   Baked Cod with Maple Mustard

Day Three

Breakfast   Poached Eggs and Salmon on Toast

Lunch   Bean Bolognese

Dinner   Chicken Quinoa Bowl

Day Four

Breakfast   Apple Cinnamon Overnight Oats

Lunch   Pomodoro Pasta with White Beans and Olives

Dinner   Mediterranean Quinoa and Halibut Bowl

Day Five

Breakfast   Buckwheat Crepes
Lunch   Chicken and Avocado Salad
Dinner   Tuna Casserole

Day Six

Breakfast   Beetroot Smoothie
Lunch   Pasta alla Erbe
Dinner   Tuna Salad Nicoise

Day Seven

Breakfast   Greek Yogurt Pancakes
Lunch   Florentine Ravioli
Dinner   Shrimp Pasta with Lemon and Garlic

Day Eight

Breakfast   Almond Honey Ricotta with Peaches
Lunch   Mini Chicken Pitas
Dinner   Beef and Blue Cheese Penne with Pesto

Day Nine
Breakfast   Muesli Scones
Lunch   Chicken and Farro Salad
Dinner   Beef Barley Soup

Day Ten
Breakfast   Gingerbread Quinoa Bake with Bananas
Lunch   Greek Fattoush Salad
Dinner   Caprese Stuffed Portobello Mushrooms

Day Eleven
Breakfast   Chocolate Coconut Oats
Lunch   Macaroni with Sausage and Ricotta
Dinner   Lamb Stew

Day Twelve
Breakfast   Egg Muffin with Ham
Lunch   Couscous with Tuna and

Pepperoncini

Dinner   Zucchini Lasagna Rolls

Day Thirteen

Breakfast   Pineapple Smoothie

Lunch   Tuna and Roasted Pepper Pasta Salad

Dinner   Minestrone Soup

Day Fourteen

Breakfast   Carrot Cake Oats

Lunch   Stuffed Eggplant

Dinner   White Fish with Lemon Orzo

Chapter 16: The Mediterranean DASH Diet On The Go

Whenever people start a new diet, one of the things to take into consideration is how this diet will affect them when they want to go out with other people. It is quite easy to stay on the diet when staying home, but no one wants to go out to a restaurant and ruin two weeks of hard work in one gluttonous night. So, is it possible to stay true to the Mediterranean DASH Diet and still enjoy time out with friends? It definitely is, as long as a few simple things are taken into consideration.

Two things that need to be watched carefully when on this new healthy eating plan are the consumption of salts and unhealthy fats. But it is easy enough to do this when eating out if you know what to look for. We all want to enjoy a nice dinner now and then, especially when someone else cooks and cleans up afterward!

It is important on the Mediterranean DASH Diet to watch the consumption of excess salt. Restaurants like to use salt because it makes food taste better and doesn't cost much. But there measures that can be taken when eating out to help avoid most of the extra salt.

Always ask that your food be cooked without adding any salt or other ingredients that may contain salt. This includes MSG, so watch for that one. Certain cooking processes scream extra salt. If something is smoked, cured, or pickled, then it contains extra salt. Also, dishes that have or are made with broth or soy sauce will have a higher salt content. Leave the salt shaker alone. Just don't touch it. Watch for condiments that are high in salt content, such as sauces, pickles, ketchup, and mustard. And when it comes to ordering appetizers try to find ones that are based on fresh fruits and vegetables. Breaded foods have a higher salt content; it's in the breading mix.

It is also possible to limit the consumption of unhealthy fats when dining out just by being careful with what you order. Ask if the food can be prepared with olive oil or corn oil if possible, rather than the usual high-fat options such as butter. When ordering a salad ask for vinegar and oil dressing on the side, rather than having the dressing put directly on the salad. When ordering poultry or meat always trim off the extra fat when the entrée comes to the table and push it to the side. Look for healthier options for the cooking process.

Anything that is stir-fried, poached, roasted, baked, broiled, grilled, or steamed is much healthier than deep fried, or for that matter any kind of fried. Order sides to the meal to be served prepared and served without sauce or butter. And when ordering fish look for the broiled or steamed options and ask for fresh herbs for seasoning during the cooking process and lemon wedges for flavoring at the tables.

Anything on the menu can hold some sort of trap that can derail your diet, not just the entrée or the salad. Try to steer clear of the bar choices, since alcohol is very high in calories. Order the drinks that are calorie free like coffee, unsweet tea, water with lime or lemon, or a diet soda. If a fruit salad is on the menu, it is always a great choice. If it is impossible to ignore the bread, ask if there are whole grain options available, and try not to slather on the butter. Many Italian restaurants offer a plate of olive oil to dip brown bread in, and it is delicious! Healthy dessert choices would include sherbet, sorbet, or fresh fruit.

And it is never necessary to upsize anything. Restaurant portions are always huge, to begin with. Have the server bring a to-go box at the beginning of the meal and put half of your food in it for lunch tomorrow. Eat an appetizer as an entrée, or ask for the lunch portion if they will serve it for dinner. Bring along a friend for dinner and split one meal between the two of you. Just ask for an extra plate when you order.

Restaurants are usually accommodating with dietary needs and restrictions. Fast food restaurants are the places to be really careful. Try to be familiar with the chain's menu options before going. Try to stick with the grilled or broiled options as opposed to the fried options. Always order the regular size meals, or even order the children's meal. Don't fall for the upsize suggestion!

It takes a bit more work to be able to eat out when following a diet and the menu choices may not be the exact ones we are used to from our pre-diet days. But with a bit of good attention to the details of the food and some careful ordering, it will never be necessary to miss those special occasions just to be able to stick to a diet.

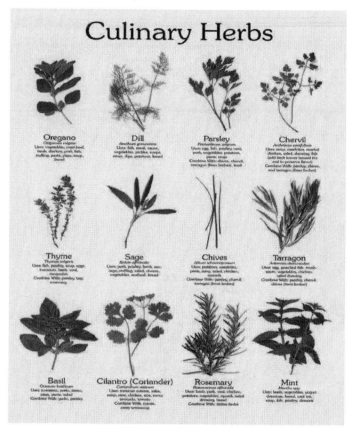

Conclusion

Thank you for making it through to the end of *DASH Diet Mediterranean Solution: The Beginner Guide for Weight Loss to Improve Health, includes Meal Prep and Delicious Recipes* by Marla Freeman. Let's hope it was informative and able to provide you with all of the tools you need to achieve your goals whatever they may be.

The next step is to clean all the bad foods out of your kitchen and stock it with wholesome, healthy foods that will get you started on your journey to a healthier lifestyle. Try all the recipes in this book and use them to make healthy menus for the entire family. Then, enjoy the new, better, healthier life you will all enjoy.

Finally, if you found this book useful in any way, a review on Amazon is always appreciated!

Made in the USA
Columbia, SC
02 January 2020